Keto Diet Snacks

Ketogenic Diet Snacks That You MUST Prepare Before Any Other!

Your Free Gifts

As a way of thanking you for the purchase, I'd like to offer you 2 complimentary gifts:

- **How To Get Through Any Weight Loss Plateau While On The Ketogenic Diet:** The title is self-explanatory; if you are struggling with getting off a weight loss plateau while on the Keto diet, you will find this free gift very eye opening on what has been ailing you. Grab your copy now by clicking/tapping here or simply enter http://bit.ly/2fantonpubketo into your browser.

- **5 Pillar Life Transformation Checklist:** This short book is about life transformation, presented in bit size pieces for easy implementation. I believe that without such a checklist, you are likely to have a hard time implementing anything in this book and any other thing you set out to do religiously and sticking to it for the long haul. It doesn't matter whether your goals relate to weight loss, relationships, personal finance, investing, personal development, improving communication in your family, your overall health, finances, improving your sex life, resolving issues in your relationship, fighting PMS successfully, investing, running a successful business, traveling etc. With a checklist like this one, you can bet that anything you do will seem a lot easier to implement until the end. Therefore, even if you don't continue reading this book, at least read the one thing that will help you in every other aspect of your life. Grab your copy [now by clicking/tapping here](http://bit.ly/2fantonfreebie) or simply enter http://bit.ly/2fantonfreebie into your browser. Your life will never be the same again (if you implement what's in this book), I promise.

PS: I'd like your feedback. If you are happy with this book, please leave a review on Amazon.

Introduction

If you've recently started following the Ketogenic diet, you know just how, at face value, the options as far as taking care of your sweet tooth and hunger, using snacks, can be pretty limited. Think about it; most times, you will hear people say you snack on nuts, eggs and something with avocado.

They rarely talk about the many other options out there as far as snacks is concerned. And if you've tried looking for snack options online, you may be overwhelmed by the sheer number of options of what you can snack on.

Lucky for you, I have sifted through all the clutter and found 50 snack recipes that will give you enough options without overwhelming your mind with options.

More precisely, this book will show you:

- Cookie recipes you can prepare
- **Fat bombs you can prepare**
- Keto balls that you can prepare
- **Ketogenic diet bars that you can prepare**
- Ketogenic diet muffins and brownies that you can prepare
- **Ketogenic diet bread recipes that you can prepare**
- Ketogenic diet crackers that you can prepare

- **Ketogenic diet nut recipes that you can prepare**
- Ketogenic diet roll up recipes that you can prepare
- **Ketogenic diet chips recipes that you can prepare**
- And much more!

If you are looking to introduce variety to your Ketogenic diet snack options, this book has 50 of them, which is just enough not to overwhelm you with options.

You won't regret it!

I hope you enjoy it!

Table of Contents

Your Free Gifts -- 2

Introduction --- 4

Tasty Ketogenic Bars --------------------------- 13

  Low Carb Granola Bars ---------------------------- 13

  Lemon Bars -- 15

  Coconut Bars -------------------------------------- 17

  Low Carb Almond Bark ------------------------------ 19

  Keto Protein Bars --------------------------------- 22

  Keto Nut Bar -------------------------------------- 24

Keto Cookies ------------------------------------- 26

  Cranberry Almond Biscotti Cookies ----------------- 26

  Homemade Thin Mints ------------------------------- 29

  Almond Flour Cookies ------------------------------ 32

  Ketogenic Chocolate No Bake Cookies --------------- 34

  Chocolate Chip Cookies ---------------------------- 37

Keto Fat Bombs ---------------------------------- 40

  Pecan Fat Bombs ----------------------------------- 40

  Macadamia Nut Fat Bombs --------------------------- 42

Chocolate Peanut Butter Fat Bomb --------------- 44

White Chocolate Fat Bombs --------------------- 46

Almond Butter Fat Bombs ----------------------- 48

Keto Balls --- 50

Sugar Free Coconut Balls ------------------------- 50

Matcha Protein Balls ----------------------------- 52

Apple Cider Donut Balls -------------------------- 54

Turmeric Coconut Balls --------------------------- 57

Chocolate Brownie Energy Balls ----------------- 59

No-Bake Brownie Balls --------------------------- 62

Keto Muffins and Brownies -------------------- 64

Avocado Brownies -------------------------------- 64

Keto Granola Brownies --------------------------- 67

Chocolate Zucchini Muffins ---------------------- 69

Keto Brownies ------------------------------------- 72

Savoury Garlic Herb Muffins -------------------- 75

Bacon Breakfast Muffins ------------------------- 77

Keto Bread Snacks ------------------------------- 79

Keto Soft Pretzel ---------------------------------- 79

Keto Croutons -- 82

Keto Bread Twists----------------------------------- 84

Keto Bread Sticks----------------------------------- 87

Keto Crackers -- 89

Keto Graham Crackers ---------------------------- 89

Keto Crackers --- 92

Keto Seed Crackers ------------------------------- 94

Keto Cheesy Crackers----------------------------- 96

Fat Head Crackers -------------------------------- 99

Keto Chips -- 101

Zucchini Chips --------------------------------------- 101

Radish Chips --- 103

Keto Cheese Chips --------------------------------- 105

Keto Salami Chips---------------------------------- 107

Keto Pepperoni Chips ----------------------------- 109

Keto Nuts-- 111

Keto Spiced Pecans-------------------------------- 111

Dill Pickle Almonds ------------------------------- 113

Almond Cranberry Trail Mix -------------------- 115

Keto Roll Up Recipes ---------------------------- 117
Hot Dogs In A Blanket --------------------------- 117

Artichoke Dip Jalapeno Poppers------------------ 119

Steak Fajita Roll-Ups---------------------------- 122

Keto Mummy Dogs --------------------------------125

Keto Cheese Roll-Ups---------------------------- 128

Conclusion --------------------------------------- 129

Do You Like My Book & Approach To Publishing?--------------------------------------- 130

1: First, I'd Love It If You Leave a Review of This Book on Amazon. --------------------------------- 130

2: Check Out My Other Keto Diet Books ------- 130

3: Let's Get In Touch----------------------------- 132

4: Grab Some Freebies On Your Way Out; Giving Is Receiving, Right? -------------------------------133

5: Suggest Topics That You'd Love Me To Cover To Increase Your Knowledge Bank. --------------133

PSS: Let Me Also Help You Save Some Money!--- 134

Copyright 2019 by Fantonpublishers.com - All rights reserved.

PS:

I have special interest in the Ketogenic diet. My wife has been following the Ketogenic diet and I can honestly say that the journey has been amazing. The diet works. And this is why I have committed to writing and publishing as many of the Ketogenic diet books as possible to give readers different options as far as the Ketogenic diet is concerned.

For instance, I have Ketogenic diet books exclusively dedicated for:

- Breakfast
- Main Meals
- Snacks
- Desserts
- Appetizers
- Soups
- Vegetarians
- Crockpot/slow cooker users
- Instant pot users
- Air fryer users
- People who are on the Paleo diet

- People who are following intermittent fasting

- People who are following carb cycling

And much more.

You can check out my [Ketogenic Diet Books fan page shop](#) for more of the books, as I continue publishing more and more. If you want me to add your category of the Ketogenic diet books that I have published so far, make sure to send me a message. I will do the heavy lifting for you and get back to you with a book that you will love.

You could also subscribe to my newsletter to receive updates whenever I have something new: http://bit.ly/2Cketodietfanton.

Tasty Ketogenic Bars

Low Carb Granola Bars

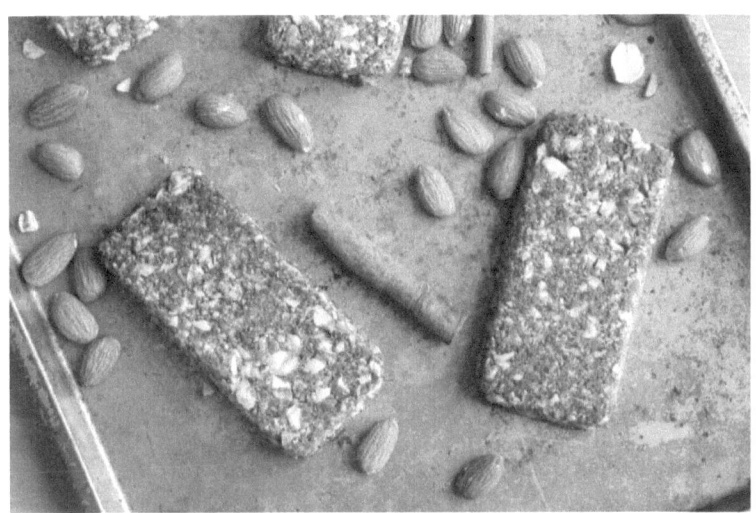

Prep time: 5 Minutes

Cook time: 30 Minutes

Total time: 50 Minutes

Servings: 4 bars

Ingredients

20 drops of liquid Stevia

½ teaspoon of vanilla extract

1 teaspoon of ground cinnamon

½ tablespoon of coconut oil

2 tablespoons of erythritol

2 tablespoons of butter powder

1 tablespoon of psyllium husk powder

1 cup of almonds, raw

Directions

Preheat the oven to around 275 degrees F then place all the ingredients in a food processor and blend for a few minutes until everything is incorporated well but you still have chunks of almonds.

Scoop the almond mixture and make a mould then using a spatula press down to form a rectangular shape.

Bake for around 30 minutes until the edges have browned then leave them to cool for about 15-20 minutes, enjoy.

Nutritional information per serving:

Calories 292, Fat 24 g, Carbs 11 g, Protein 8 g

Lemon Bars

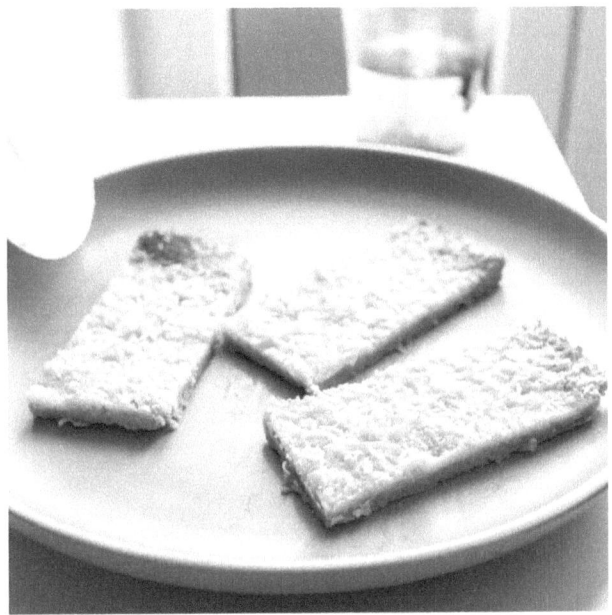

Prep time: 15 Minutes

Cook time: 30 Minutes

Total time: 45 Minutes

Servings: 16

Ingredients

For the crust

Dash of salt

2 teaspoons of vanilla extract

1 teaspoon of lemon juice

1/3 cup of ghee

2 cups of almond flour

Filling

Lemon zest to be used as topping

Dash of salt

1 tablespoon of coconut flour

½ cup of Stevia

6 tablespoons of ghee

6 egg yolks

½ cup of lemon juice

Directions

Preheat the oven to about 350 degrees F or 175 degrees C then mix the crust ingredients. Press the mixture into the bottom part of a baking pan. Bake for around 10 minutes.

Mix the filling ingredients and pour over the crust. Bake again for another 15-20 minutes until it sets. Leave to cool and then garnish with lemon zest.

Nutritional information per serving:

Calories 170, Fat 17g, Carbs 3g, Protein 2g

Coconut Bars

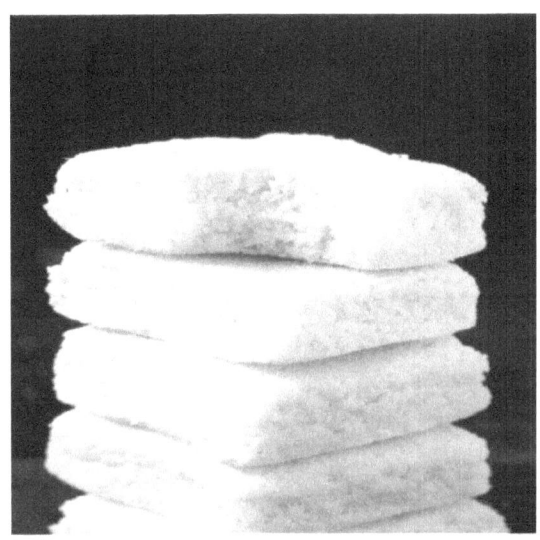

Prep time: 2 Minutes

Cook time: 3 Minutes

Total time: 5 Minutes

Servings: 20

Ingredients

¼ cup of monk-fruit sweetened maple syrup

1 cup of melted coconut oil

3 cups of coconut flakes, shredded and unsweetened

Directions

Coat an 8*10 inch baking pan with some parchment paper and set aside; you can also use a loaf pan.

In a bowl put in the coconut then add in maple syrup and coconut oil and mix well. If the mixture is very crumbly, you add in more syrup or water.

Pour the mixture into the coated pan and place in the refrigerator until it becomes firm. Once ready, slice into squares and bon a petite.

Nutritional information per serving:

Calories 108, Fat 11g, Carbs 2g, Protein 2g

Low Carb Almond Bark

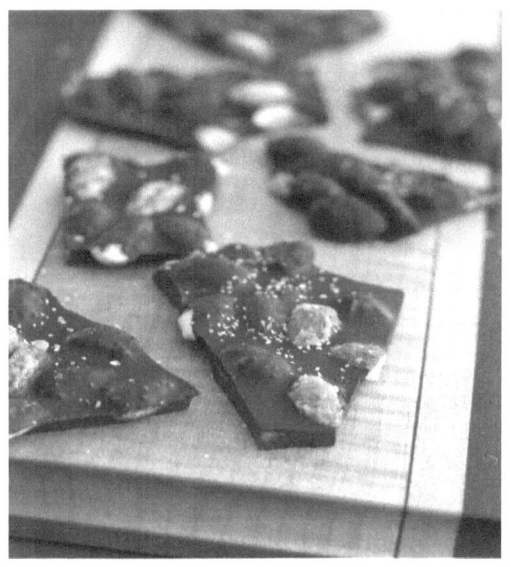

Prep time: 10 Minutes

Cook time: 15 Minutes

Total time: 25 Minutes

Servings: 20 barks

Ingredients

½ teaspoon of vanilla extract

¾ cup of cocoa powder

½ cup of swerve sweetener, powdered and sifted

2 ½ ounces of copped chocolate, unsweetened

4 ounces of cocoa butter

¼ teaspoon of sea salt

1 ½ cups of unsalted almonds, roasted

1 tablespoon of butter

2 tablespoons of water

½ cup of swerve sweetener

Sea salt to be used for sprinkling

Directions

Coat a baking dish with some parchment paper.

Mix the water with the swerve and stir over moderate heat in a pan. Let the mixture cook for about seven to nine minutes until it darkens.

Whisk butter into the mixture and remove the pan from heat, put in almonds and mix quickly to coat then add salt and mix.

Place the almonds in the baking dish and spread them making sure to break up clumps.

Melt chocolate together with cocoa butter until smooth in a heavy pan over low heat. Mix in erythritol powder, then add in cocoa powder and combine until smooth.

Remove the pan from heat and mix in vanilla extract. Put aside ¼ cup of almonds then mix the rest of almonds with chocolate. Spread the mixture onto the baking dish making sure to keep the nuts in one layer then sprinkle on top the reserved almonds and some sea salt.

Place the mixture in a fridge for around 3 hours until it sets then break into big chunks using your hands.

Nutritional information per serving:

Calories 144, Carbs 5g, Fat 14g, Protein 3g

Keto Protein Bars

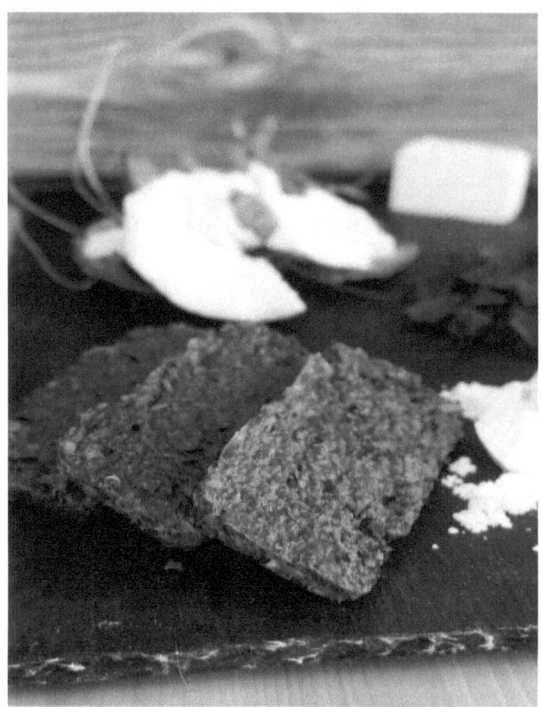

Prep time: 10 Minutes

Cooking time: 20 Minutes

Total time: 30 Minutes

Ingredients

35 drops of liquid Stevia

18 grams of erythritol

¾ tablespoon of heavy whipping cream

1 ½ tablespoons of water

2 ¼ tablespoons of butter

23 grams of protein powder, unflavored

130 grams of bakers chocolate, unsweetened

150 grams of coconut meat, raw

Directions

Mix all of the ingredients in a blender and blend well ensuring that you scrape the sides of the blender often.

Pour the batter onto parchment paper and make 6 bars.

Bake the bars in the oven at about 250 degrees C for around 20 minutes.

Once ready, let then cool and enjoy. You can store the bars in the fridge for up to 3 weeks.

Nutritional information per serving:

Calories 278, Fat 23 g, Carbs 9.8 g, Protein 7.5 g

Keto Nut Bar

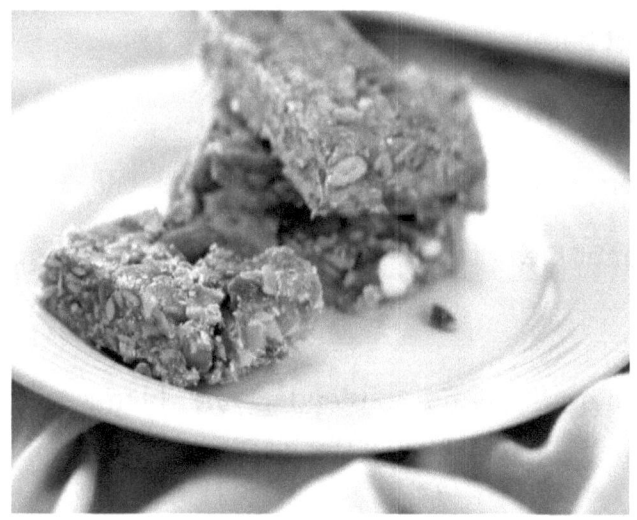

Prep time: 1 Hour 10 Minutes

Cook time: 0 Minutes

Total time: 1 Hour 10 Minutes

Servings: 10 Bars

Ingredients

1/3 cup of fibre syrup

3 tablespoons of almond butter

1 teaspoon of vanilla essence

2 tablespoons of coconut oil

¼ teaspoon of salt

1 tablespoon of chia seeds

½ cup of desiccated coconut

2 cups of mixed nuts, sunflower seeds, pumpkin seeds

Directions

Coat 20cm square tin with baking paper then oil it a little bit.

Chop roughly the bigger nuts then in a bowl mix salt, chia seeds and desiccated coconut. Combine fibre syrup, almond butter, vanilla, and coconut oil in a bowl that is microwave safe.

Microwave butter and oil for about 30 seconds and stir until well combined. Drizzle this over the seeds and nuts, mix thoroughly.

Put in the fridge for around an hour then cut into bars and enjoy.

Nutritional information per serving:

Calories 268, Fat 22g, Carbs 15 g, Protein 7 g

Keto Cookies

Cranberry Almond Biscotti Cookies

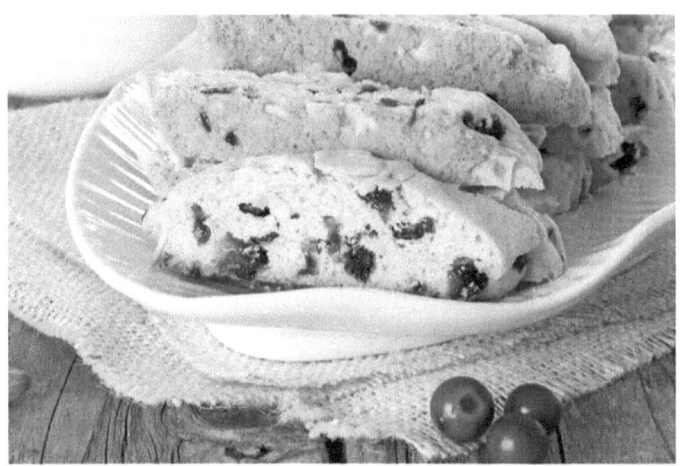

Prep time: 5 Minutes

Cook time: 40 Minutes

Total time: 45 Minutes

Servings: 14

Ingredients

½ cup of almonds, sliced

½ cup of dried cranberries, sugar fee

¼ teaspoon of salt

½ teaspoon of baking soda

¼ cup of coconut flour

1 ½ cups of almond flour

¼ teaspoon of stevia

1/3 cup of sweetener, low carb

1 teaspoon of vanilla

2 eggs

Dark chocolate, low carb, melted

Directions

Whisk together in an electric mixer Stevia, swerve, vanilla and eggs until frothy.

In another bowl mix salt, baking soda, coconut flour and almond flour then add the flour mixture into the egg mixture and mix well until you make a dough then add in almonds and cranberries.

On a cookie dish coated with some parchment paper, make a rectangle shape from the dough then bake for around 20 minutes at 350 degrees F or until it browns.

Transfer to a platter and let it completely cool. Diagonally cut the dough into thin slices then put each piece onto a coated baking dish. Bake for around 15-20 minutes at 350 degrees F until well toasted.

Let them cool then sprinkle with some melted chocolate, if you like.

Keto Diet Snacks

Nutritional information per serving:

Calories 112, Fat 9 g, Carbs 6 g, Protein 5 g

Homemade Thin Mints

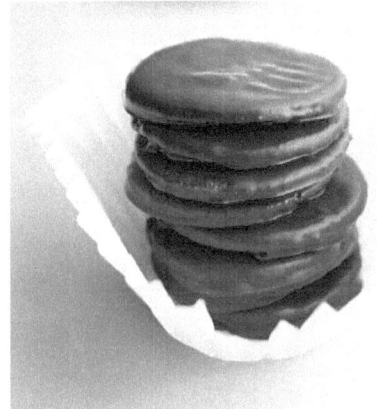

Prep time: 30 Minutes

Cook time: 30 Minutes

Total time: 1 hour

Servings: 20

Ingredients

Cookies

1/8 teaspoon of liquid Stevia extract

½ teaspoon of vanilla extract

2 tablespoons of melted butter

1 egg, beaten slightly

¼ teaspoon of salt

1 teaspoon of baking powder

¼ cup of swerve sweetener

1/3 cup of cocoa powder

1 ¾ cups of almond flour

Coating

1 teaspoon of peppermint extract

7 ounces of dark chocolate, sugar free

1 tablespoon of coconut oil

Directions

To make the cookies:

Preheat oven to around 300 degrees F then coat 2 baking dishes with some parchment paper.

In a mixing bowl mix salt, baking powder, sweetener, cacao powder and almond flour, and then add in Stevia, vanilla, butter and egg. Mix well until you have a dough.

Place the dough between two sheets of parchment paper and roll it out to around 1/8 inch thick. Remove the top sheet of parchment paper, put aside then with a cookie slicer slice out the dough into circles and gently lift them.

Put the cut out circles on the baking dish and roll again the dough. Repeat the same until you have very little dough left.

Bake the cookies for around 30 minutes until firm then remove from the oven and leave them to cool for a few minutes.

To make the coating:

Put metal bowl on top of a dish over medium heat with some water that is simmering gently, making sure the water does not get into the bowl.

Place the chocolate and butter into the bowl and melt for a few minutes until the mixture is smooth; make sure you stir frequently. Remove the bowl from the heat then add in the peppermint extract.

Put the cookie into the butter and chocolate mixture and turn them to the other side making sure to coat well the cookies. Pass gently the coated cookie in between forks to get rid of the excess chocolate mixture then put the cookies on some waxed paper for them to set, enjoy.

Nutritional information per serving:

Calories 116, Fat 10.41 g, Carbs 6.99 g, Protein 3.08 g

Almond Flour Cookies

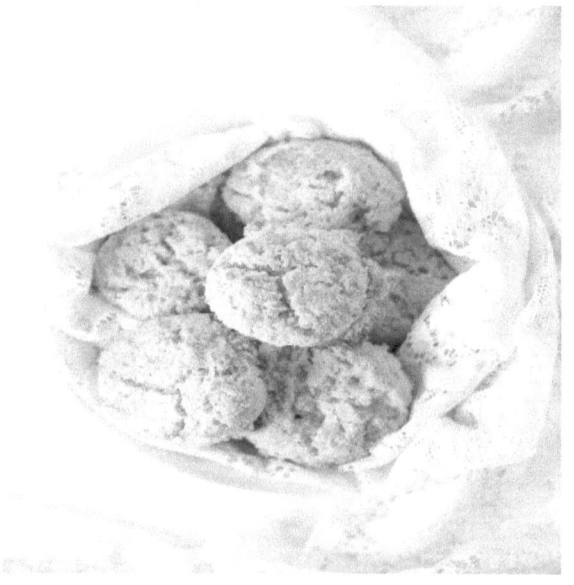

Prep time: 10 Minutes

Cook time: 15 Minutes

Total time: 25 Minutes

Servings: 12 biscuits

Ingredients

1/3 cup of butter, melted

2 large eggs, beaten

½ teaspoon of sea salt

2 teaspoons of baking powder, gluten free

2 cups of almond flour, blanched

Directions

Preheat the oven to about 350 degrees F then coat baking dish with some parchment paper.

Combine all the dry ingredients in a mixing bowl then add in the remaining ingredients.

With a spoon, scoop the dough and place on the coated baking dish then make into biscuits.

Repeat until all the dough is finished then bake for around 15 minutes until golden and firm. Place on a cooling rack to cool then once cooled enjoy.

Nutritional information per serving:

Calories 164, Fat 15g, Protein 5g, Carbs 4g

Ketogenic Chocolate No Bake Cookies

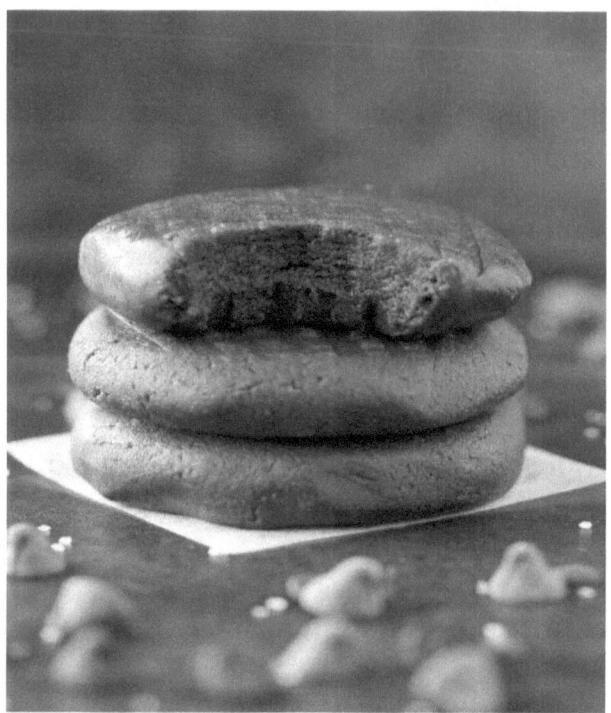

Prep time: 5 Minutes

Cook time: 0 Minutes

Total time: 5 Minutes

Servings: 20 cookies

Ingredients

¾ cup of coconut flour

½ cup of Swerve

2 cups of Low Carb Nutella

Directions

Line a plate with some parchment paper and put aside.

In a bowl, mix coconut flour, swerve and Nutella. Mix well until a thick mixture is formed.

Form small balls from the dough using clean hands then press to form a cookie like shape and place them on the coated plate. Place the cookies in the refrigerator until firm.

Nutritional information per serving:

Calories 98, Fat 8 g, Carbs 5 g, Protein 4 g

Low Carb Nutella

Ingredients

¼ cup coconut oil

½ cup cocoa powder

1 cup granulated sweetener

4 cups raw unsalted hazelnuts

Directions

Preheat the oven to 350 degrees F.

Use parchment paper to line a baking tray. Spread the hazelnuts on the try and roast until golden brown or for around 10 minutes.

Remove the skins from the hazelnuts then put the hazelnuts into a food processor and pulse until you have a paste-like consistency.

Once you have smooth batter add in the other ingredients and blend until creamy and smooth. If too thick, you can add in some coconut oil.

Chocolate Chip Cookies

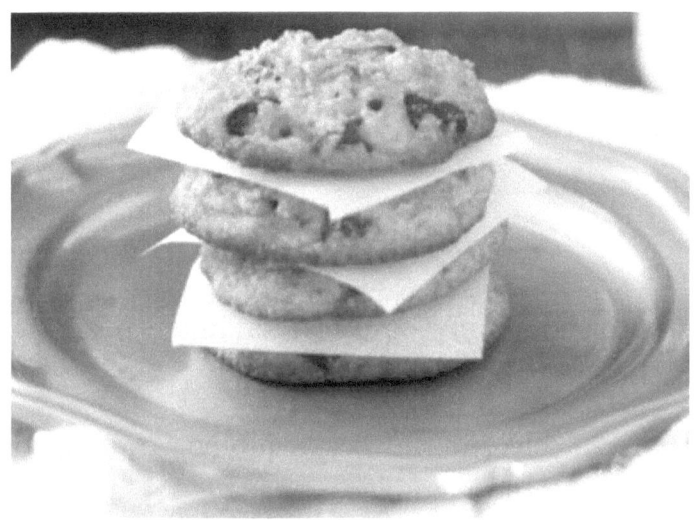

Prep time: 10 Minutes

Cook time: 20 Minutes

Total time: 30 Minutes

Servings: 24

Ingredients

½ cup of sugar free chocolate chips

1 large egg

½ teaspoon of vanilla extract

5 ½ tablespoons of cold butter

2/3 cup of swerve sweetener

1/8 teaspoon of sea salt

1 ½ teaspoons of baking powder

1 tablespoon of coconut flour

1 ¼ cups of almond flour

Directions

Preheat the oven to about 325 degrees F then line two baking sheets with parchment paper.

In the bowl of an electric mixer, combine granulated sweetener and butter until well mixed.

Add in vanilla extract and egg and mix again until well combined then in another bowl mix together sea salt, baking powder, coconut flour and almond flour. Add dry ingredients to wet ingredients and mix well. Fold in the pecans and chocolate chips.

Put around one tablespoon of the dough on the baking dish and make into a cookie. Repeat this until all the dough has been used up. Make sure that the cookies are one and a half inches away from each other on the baking sheet.

Bake for about 12-15 minutes until the cookies turn brown at the bottom. Remove the cookies from the oven, cool them for 25 minutes until the cookies are set, and firm.

Nutritional information per serving:

Keto Diet Snacks

Calories 90, Fat 8 g, Carbs 3 g, Protein 2 g

Keto Fat Bombs

Pecan Fat Bombs

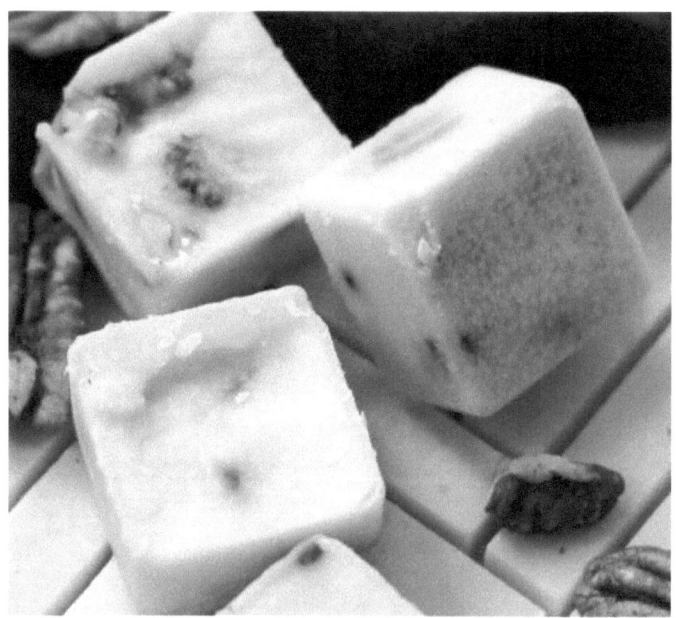

Prep time: 2 Minutes

Cook time: 5 Minutes

Total time: 7 Minutes

Servings: 12 Fat bombs

Ingredients

7-8 drops of stevia

1/8 teaspoon of sea salt

½ teaspoon of vanilla extract

¼ cup of coconut oil

¼ cup of butter

¼ cup of coconut butter

½ cup of pecans

Directions

Put a pan over medium heat and then add in the pecans and toast them as you stir frequently. When the pecans turn dark and start smelling toasty transfer to a dish. Once cooled, slice the pecans into big pieces.

In a pan over low heat, mix coconut oil, ghee and coconut butter until it melts. Once melted, add in the sweetener, salt and vanilla extract and remove from heat.

Divide the pecans into a silicon mould with several cubes. Pour the coconut butter mixture over the pecans and put in the freezer for around thirty minutes so that the fat bombs become hard.

Nutritional information per serving:

Calories 145, Fat 16g, Protein 1g, Carbs 2g

Macadamia Nut Fat Bombs

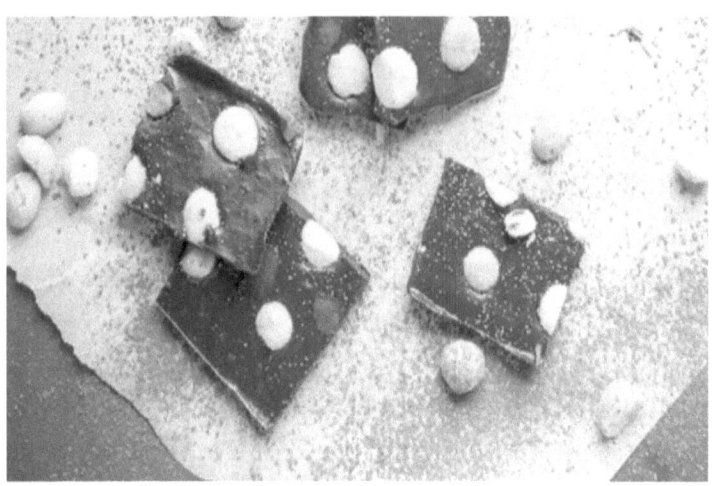

Prep time: 20 Minutes

Cook time: 20 Minutes

Total time: 40 Minutes

Servings: 6

Ingredients

Pinch of salt

12 macadamia nuts

1 teaspoon of vanilla extract

2 tablespoons of erythritol

2 tablespoons of unsweetened cocoa powder

1/3 cup of coconut oil, unrefined

Directions

Mix in a medium bowl, vanilla extract, sweetener, cocoa powder and coconut oil until the mixture is smooth.

Line a container with some parchment paper then add in vanilla mixture and with a spatula spread evenly the mixture.

Sprinkle the nuts and some salt on top. Store in the freezer overnight and enjoy.

Nutritional information per serving:

Calories 99, Fat 16.9 g, Carbs 1.9 g, Protein 0.8 g

Keto Diet Snacks

Chocolate Peanut Butter Fat Bomb

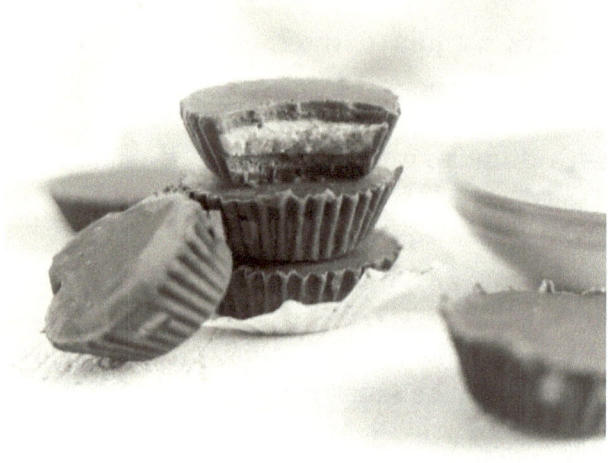

Prep time: 1 Minute

Cook time: 10 Minutes

Total time: 11 Minutes

Servings: 12 fat bombs

Ingredients

½ teaspoon of vanilla Stevia drops

1 tablespoon of cocoa

1 ounce of baking chocolate, unsweetened

¼ cup of coconut oil

¼ cup of peanut butter with no sugar

Directions

Melt the cocoa, baking chocolate, coconut oil and peanut butter in a skillet over medium heat.

Remove the mixture from the heat then mix in Stevia. Pour the cocoa mixture in moulds and freeze until they become hard.

Remove fat bombs from the moulds and enjoy. You can store the remaining fat bombs in a dish that is airtight.

Nutritional information per serving:

Calories 88, Fat 8.7 g, Carbs 2.2 g, Protein 1.7 g

White Chocolate Fat Bombs

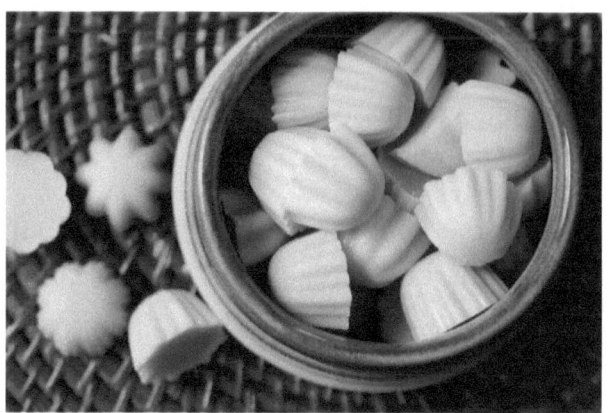

Prep time: 5 Minutes

Cook time: 10 Minutes

Total time: 15 Minutes

Servings: 8

Ingredients

10 drops of Stevia drops, vanilla

¼ cup of coconut oil

¼ cup of cocoa butter

Directions

In a skillet on low heat melt coconut oil and cocoa butter, and then mix well until combined.

Remove skillet from the heat and mix in Stevia then pour the mixture into silicone moulds.

Place the moulds in the freezer until hard then remove from the freezer and store the remaining bombs in the fridge.

Nutritional information per serving:

Calories 125, Fat 10 g, Carbs 0 g, Protein 0 g

Almond Butter Fat Bombs

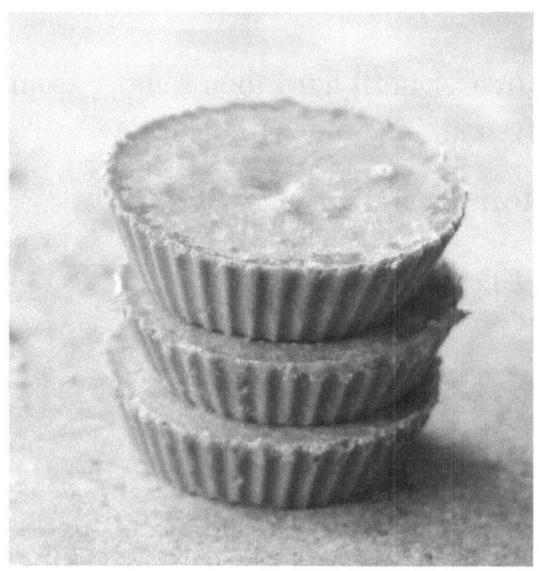

Prep time: 5 Minutes

Cooking time: 5 Minutes

Total time: 10 Minutes

Servings: 6 Fat bombs

Ingredients

¼ cup of erythritol

2 tablespoons of cacao powder

¼ cup of unrefined coconut oil

¼ cup of almond butter

Directions

Add coconut oil and almond butter into a microwave-safe bowl and microwave for about 30-45 seconds until melted then mix until the mixture is smooth.

Mix in cacao powder and erythritol then pour the mixture into moulds and place in the freezer until firm.

Nutritional information per serving:

Calories 189, Fat 19.1 g, Carbs 3.6 g, Protein 3.2 g

Keto Balls

Sugar Free Coconut Balls

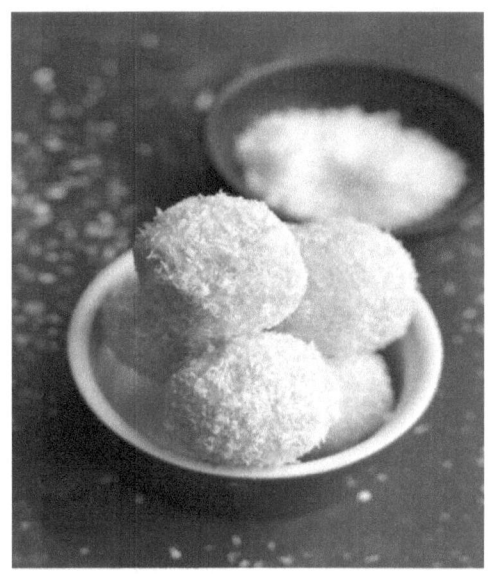

Prep time: 40 Minutes

Cook time: 5 Minutes

Total time: 45 Minutes

Servings: 12 balls

Ingredients

Stevia powder to taste

½ teaspoon of cinnamon, ground

1 cup of shredded coconut, unsweetened

1 cup of coconut butter

Directions

Put Stevia, cinnamon and coconut butter in a bowl over double broiler. Heat until the ingredients are soft.

Put the bowl into the fridge for about twenty minutes, and then remove and roll the mixture into twelve balls.

Return the balls in the fridge for twenty minutes to set, put coconut flakes on a tray then sprinkle them over the balls. You can store the balls in the fridge up to two weeks.

Nutritional information per serving:

Calories 196, Protein 2 g, Fat 18 g, Carbs 6 g

Matcha Protein Balls

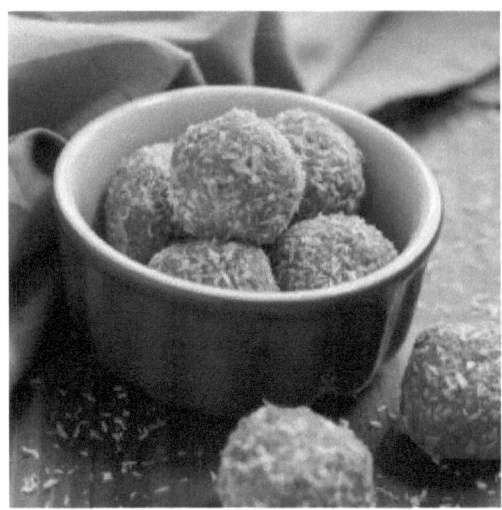

Prep time: 10 Minutes

Cook time: 0 Minutes

Total time: 10 Minutes

Servings: 7 balls

Ingredients

1 tablespoon of shredded coconut, unsweetened and dried

A pinch of salt

1 tablespoon of coconut oil

15 drops of liquid Stevia

1 packet of vital proteins Matcha collagen

¼ cup of unsweetened and dried coconut, shredded

¼ cup of almond butter

Directions

Combine in a food processor coconut oil, Stevia, Matcha collagen, dried coconut and almond butter. Mix in salt and then blend until the mixture is smooth.

Scoop the mixture using a spoon and make balls from it. If the mixture is too soft, you can put in the freezer until it becomes firm to be able to make balls from it. Roll the balls in the extra coconut and enjoy.

Nutritional information per serving:

Calories 116, Fat 9 g, Carbs 3 g, Protein 5 g

Apple Cider Donut Balls

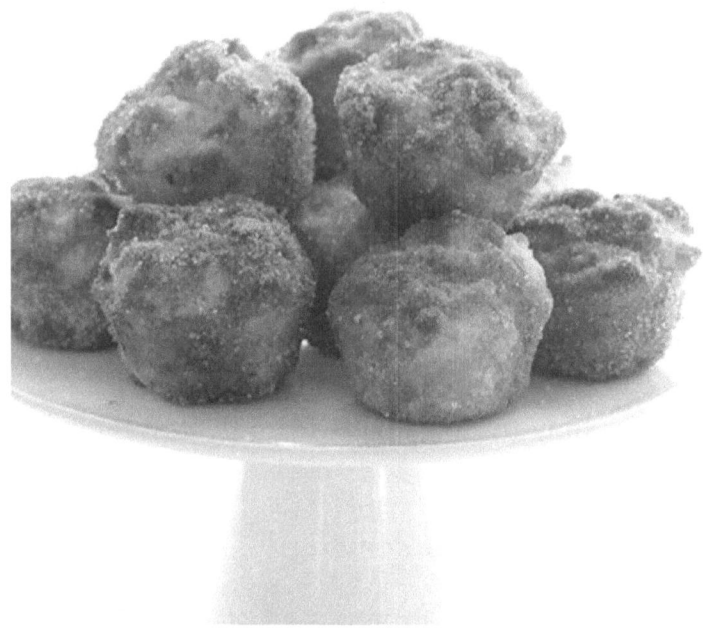

Prep time: 10 Minutes

Cook time: 20 Minutes

Total time: 30 Minutes

Servings: 12

Ingredients

Donut bites

1 ½ teaspoons of apple extract

1 ½ tablespoons of apple cider vinegar

¼ cup of melted butter

1/3 cup of water

2 eggs, large

½ teaspoon of salt

½ teaspoon of cinnamon

2 teaspoons of baking powder

¼ cup of whey protein powder, unflavored

½ cup of swerve sweetener

2 cups of almond flour

Coating

¼ cup of melted butter

1 to 2 teaspoons of cinnamon

¼ cup of swerve sweetener

Directions

Preheat the oven to about 325 degrees F then with some oil grease a muffin tin.

In a bowl, mix salt, cinnamon, baking powder, protein powder, sweetener and almond flour. Add in apple extract, apple cider vinegar, butter, water and eggs, mix well.

Pour the batter into the muffin tin and bake for about fifteen to twenty minutes until the muffins are firm.

Remove the muffin tin from the oven and let the muffins cool for about ten minutes then move them to a rack to completely cool.

In a bowl mix cinnamon and sweetener, dip the donuts in the melted butter to coat. Roll the donuts in the sweetener and cinnamon mix.

Nutritional information per serving:

Calories 164, Fat 13.71 g, Carbs 4.81 g, Proteins 6.52 g

Turmeric Coconut Balls

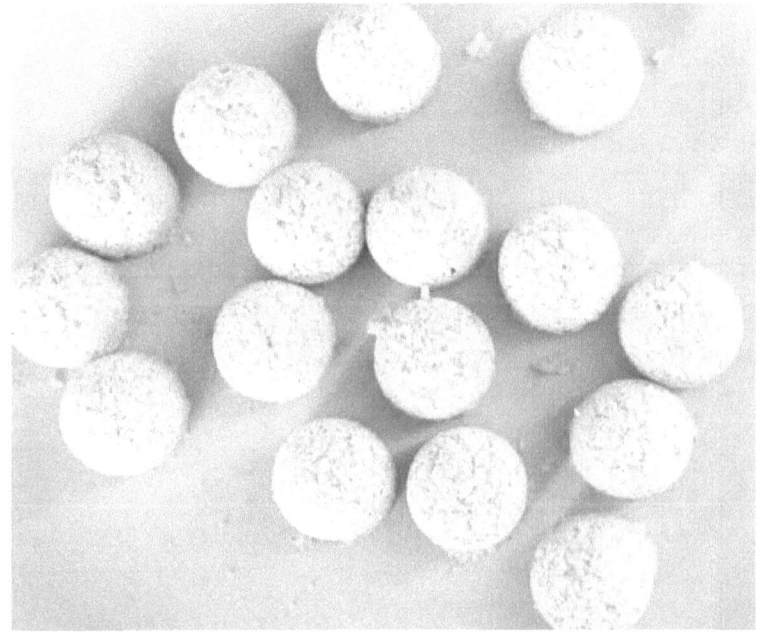

Prep time: 10 Minutes

Cook time: 0 Minutes

Total time: 10 Minutes

Servings: 15

Ingredients

Erythritol to taste

1 tablespoon of turmeric powder

½ cup of coconut butter

1 cup of shredded coconut, unsweetened

Directions

Slightly melt coconut butter then mix all the ingredients. You can adjust the taste to fit your liking and make sure that the mixture is not very crumbly. You can add in some coconut oil if it is too crumbly.

Make balls from the mixture and place on a platter. Put in the freezer for around 2 hours until they set.

Nutritional information per serving:

Calories 93, Fat 8g, Carbs 3g, Protein 1g

Chocolate Brownie Energy Balls

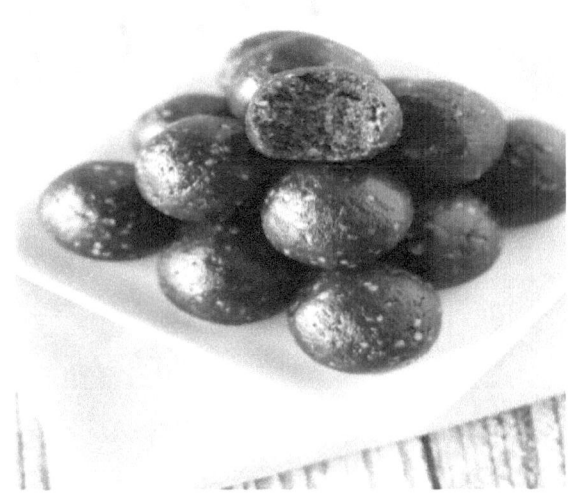

Prep time: 10 Minutes

Cook time: 20 Minutes

Total time: 30 Minutes

Servings: 24 bites

Ingredients

Chocolate coating

1 tablespoon of butter

4 ounces of dark chocolate, sugar free

Energy bites

2 tablespoons of coconut flour

1/3 cup of walnuts, copped

½ cup of protein powder, unflavored

1 cup of coconut, shredded

1 cup of almond flour

1 lightly beaten egg

1/3 cup of swerve sweetener

1/3 cup of cocoa powder, unsweetened

½ cup butter

Directions

To make balls:

Line a baking dish with some waxed or parchment paper then in a skillet over low heat, melt coconut oil and butter.

Mix in sweetener and cocoa powder then add in egg and mix well. Cook for around 5 minutes on low heat then remove from the heat.

In a mixing bowl, combine coconut flour, chopped nuts, protein powder, shredded coconut and almond flour. Combine the mixture until well mixed.

Scoop out the mixture and make into balls using clean hands then put on the lined baking sheet. Place the baking sheet in the fridge for the balls to set.

To make coating:

Put a mixing or metal bowl on a pan of water that is simmering gently ensuring that water does not get into the bowl.

Add into the bowl, butter and chocolate and melt. Dip the bites into the chocolate mixture to coat them. With a fork, gently lift the bite and tap the fork at the side of mixing bowl to get rid of the excess chocolate.

Put the bites on baking dish lined with waxed paper then leave to set and enjoy.

Nutritional information per serving:

Calories 179, Fat 16.47 g, Carbs 6.56 g, Protein 4.2 g

No-Bake Brownie Balls

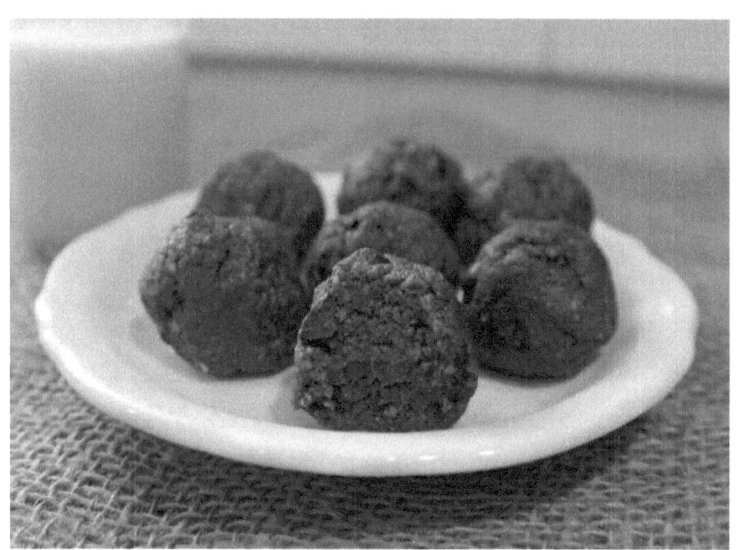

Prep time: 15 Minutes

Cook time: 0 Minutes

Total time: 35 Minutes

Servings: 18

Ingredients

½ teaspoon of pure vanilla

¼ cup of dark chocolate chips

2 tablespoons of coconut flour

¼ cup of swerve

½ cup of peanut butter

¼ cup of cocoa powder

1/8 teaspoon of sea salt

1 cup of walnuts, whole

Directions

Place salt and walnuts in a food processor and process until fine. Add swerve, vanilla, peanut butter and cocoa powder, and process until batter comes together and is well mixed.

You can add coconut flour depending on how thick the peanut butter is. If adding coconut flour, add 1 tablespoon each time and mix until it is well combined and you get the desired consistency. If you may have added too much coconut flour, just put in a splash of milk. Add in the chocolate chips and mix.

Line a baking sheet with some parchment paper. Make small balls using the dough and place them on the parchment paper.

Put baking dish in the fridge and freeze for 10 to 20 minutes or until they are firm. Enjoy and store the remaining cookies in a container and place in the fridge.

Nutritional information per serving:

Calories 110, Fat 9 g, Carbs 5 g, Protein 3 g

Keto Muffins and Brownies

Avocado Brownies

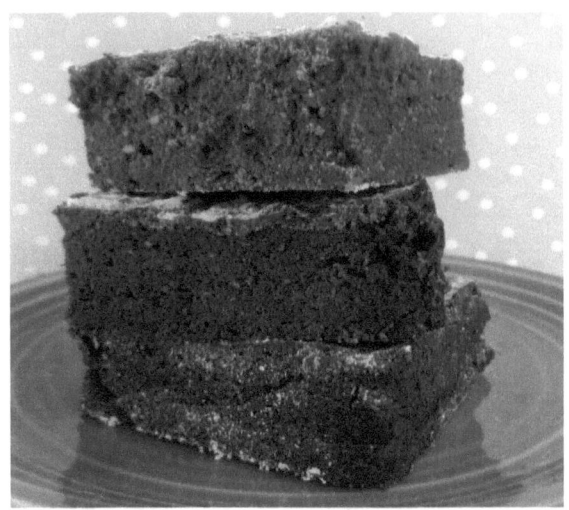

Prep time: 10 Minutes

Cook time: 35 Minutes

Total time: 45 Minutes

Servings: 12 pieces

Ingredients

Dry ingredients

¼ cup of erythritol

¼ teaspoon of salt

1 teaspoon of baking powder

¼ teaspoon of baking soda

90 grams of almond flour, blanched

Other ingredients

100 grams of melted dark chocolate

2 eggs

3 tablespoons of coconut oil

1 teaspoon of Stevia powder

4 tablespoons of cocoa powder

½ teaspoon of vanilla

250 grams of avocado

Directions

Preheat the oven to 350 degrees F then peel avocados, remove pit and put in the food processor. Pulse until the mixture is smooth then add in the other ingredients apart from the dry ones, ensuring you pulse for a couple of seconds each time you add an ingredient.

In another bowl mix the dry ingredients ensuring you mix well then add into food processor. Mix until well combined.

Line a baking pan preferably a 30*20 cm with parchment paper. Pour the batter on top and evenly spread it then put in the oven.

Bake for around 35 minutes then leave it to cool and cut into twelve pieces.

Nutritional information per serving:

Calories 158, Fat 14.29 g, Carbs 9.01 g, Protein 3.84 g

Keto Granola Brownies

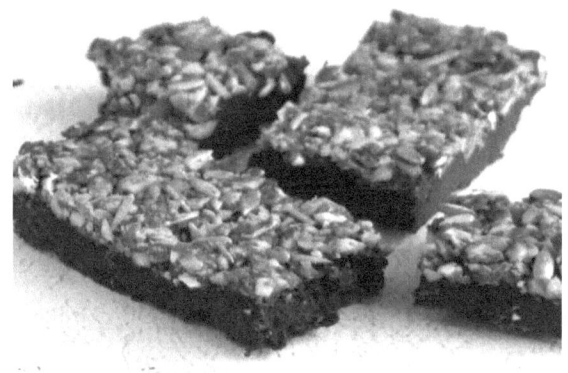

Prep time: 20 Minutes

Cook time: 18 Minutes

Total time: 38 Minutes

Servings: 9

Ingredients

1 cup of nuts and seeds for topping

½ cup of cacao powder, unsweetened

Dash of Stevia

¼ cup of erythritol

1 cup of almond flour

1/3 cup of coconut cream, warmed

2 teaspoon of vanilla extract

3 whisked eggs, large

¼ cup of coconut oil, warmed

Directions

Preheat the oven to around 175 degrees C or 350 degrees F then melt coconut oil and put aside. Mix coconut cream, vanilla extract and eggs then once the coconut oil has cooled, stir into the egg mixture.

In another bowl, mix well Stevia, erythritol and almond flour then add the egg mixture into the flour mixture. Mix well then add the mixture into a greased baking sheet about 6*6 inches. Sprinkle the seeds and nuts over the mixture and spread out until distributed evenly.

Using your hands, press down the granola into the mixture to make sure you have an intact topping.

Bake for around 15-18 minutes, remove from the oven and put aside to completely cool. Slice into squares or the shape you want, enjoy.

Nutritional information per serving:

Calories 258, Fat 24 g, Carbs 7 g, Protein 8 g

Chocolate Zucchini Muffins

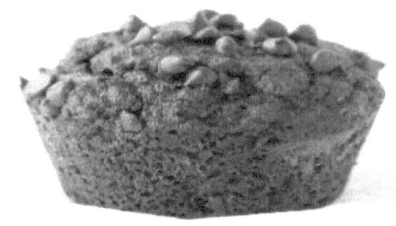

Prep time: 15 Minutes

Cook time: 15 Minutes

Total time: 30 Minutes

Servings: 10 muffins

Ingredients

Wet ingredients

¼ cup of chocolate chips, sugar free

½ teaspoon of Stevia glyceride

½ teaspoon of vanilla

6 large eggs

Dry Ingredients

5 ounces of zucchini

¼ teaspoon of salt

¼ teaspoon of xanthan gum

½ teaspoon of instant coffee granules

1 tablespoon of baking powder

¼ cup of cocoa powder

½ cup of granulated swerve

¾ cup of coconut flour

Melt together ingredients

1 ounce baking chocolate, unsweetened

4 ounces of ghee

Directions

Preheat the oven to about 350 degrees F then position a rack at the centre of oven.

Coat 10 holes of a medium muffin tin with some baking spray.

Grate the zucchini, put in a colander and sprinkle with some salt. Thoroughly mix and leave the zucchini to sit for a few minutes.

Cut the unsweetened baking chocolate finely then measure out dry ingredients in a mixing bowl and mix them well together. Make sure to break up lumps if any.

In a dish, that is microwave safe, melt baking chocolate and butter at around 30 seconds time intervals.

Pour wet ingredients into dry mixture ensuring you start with eggs. Mix until well combined then add in the butter and chocolate mixture; combine until everything is well incorporated. Using your hands, squeeze out excess water from the zucchini and then add them into the bowl and mix.

Scoop the batter into the muffin holes. Lift muffin tin from the counter and tap on the counter to ensure the batter settles well in the muffin hole. Sprinkle some chocolate chips on top and bake for around 15-18 minutes, checking the muffins at about 12 minutes to avoid over baking them.

Once ready, remove from oven and leave them to cool on the rack for around 3 minutes before serving.

Nutritional information per serving:

Calories 203, Fat 17 g, Carbs 9 g, Protein 6 g

Keto Brownies

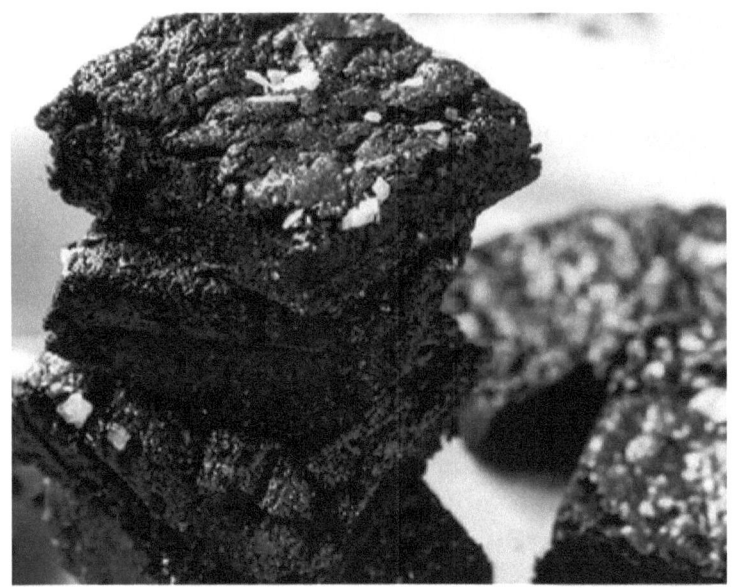

Prep time: 15 minutes

Cook time: 20 Minutes

Total time: 35 Minutes

Servings: 16

Ingredients

Flaky sea salt

70 grams of almond flour

2 eggs, room temp

½ teaspoon of kosher salt

80 grams of cocoa powder

140-200 grams of powdered erythritol

8 tablespoons of coconut oil

Directions

Place a rack at the bottom 3rd of the oven then preheat to about 350 degrees F or 180 degrees Celsius.

Line the sides and bottom part of a baking dish with some parchment paper and put aside.

In a small heatproof bowl mix salt, cocoa powder, sweetener and butter. Melt the mixture in a water bath. Heat the mixture until almost all of the sweetener has melted and is well combined. Most of the erythritol will not dissolve, take off from heat and allow to cool.

Mix each egg at a time until the mixture is well combined; the mixture should be smooth and the sweetener dissolved in it. When using erythritol and batter becomes thick you can add an extra egg, but do not mix too much as your brownies may appear cakey instead of fudgy. Mix in the almond flour vigorously until well combined.

Pour into the baking sheet and place in the oven. Bake for about 15 to 25 minutes or until when a toothpick is inserted in the centre, it comes out dry. This varies depending with the oven; keep on checking from time to time, as your brownies will cook as they cool.

Sprinkle with some salt and let the brownie cool on a cooling rack. Once cooled enough to handle, lift the brownie using the ends of the parchment paper and slice accordingly.

Nutritional information per serving:

Calories 102, Fat 9 g, Carbs 3 g, Protein 2 g

Savoury Garlic Herb Muffins

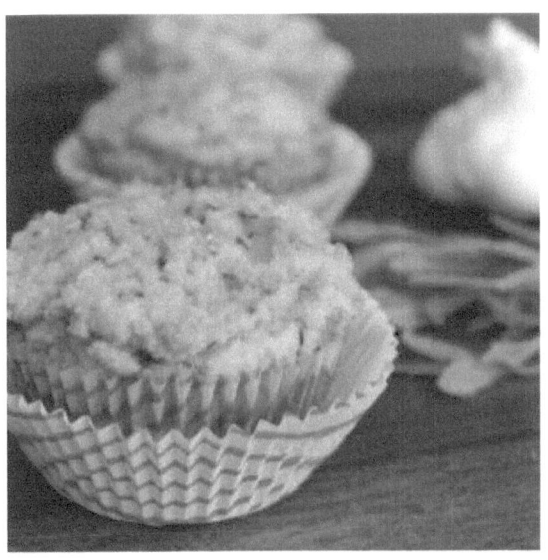

Prep time: 10 Minutes

Cook time: 30 Minutes

Total time: 40 Minutes

Servings: 8 Muffins

Ingredients

½ teaspoon of sage

½ teaspoon of thyme

½ teaspoon of rosemary

1 teaspoon of garlic powder

1 teaspoon of apple cider vinegar

4 pasture eggs

½ cup and 2 tablespoons of coconut milk

¼ cup of coconut oil

½ to 1 teaspoon of sea salt

1 teaspoon of baking soda

½ cup of coconut flour

Directions

Preheat the oven to about 350 degrees F then melt coconut oil.

Once melted, mix the coconut oil with the remaining ingredients.

Add batter in muffin tin lined with muffin liners, ensuring that you fill them ¾ full as muffins begin to rise up when ready.

Place in the oven for about 20 to 30 minutes or until browned slightly.

Nutritional information per serving:

Calories 160, Fat 13 g, Carbs 5 g, Protein 4 g

Bacon Breakfast Muffins

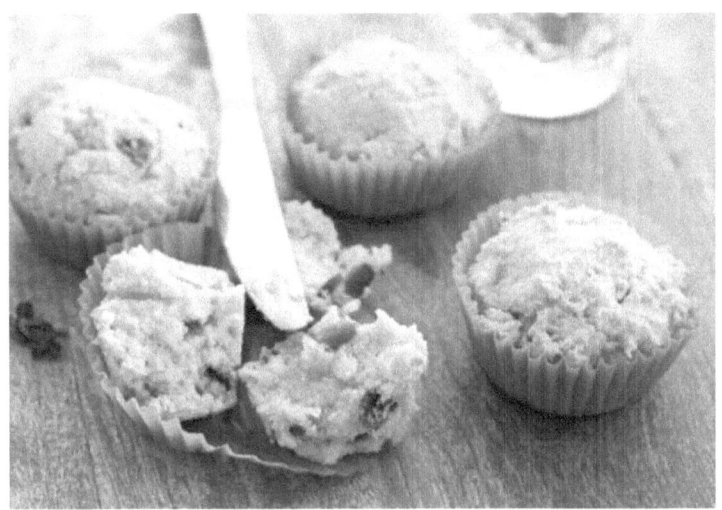

Prep time: 10 Minutes

Cook time: 20 Minutes

Total time: 30 Minutes

Servings: 12 Muffins

Ingredients

½ teaspoon of salt

1 teaspoon of baking soda

2 teaspoons of lemon thyme

4 eggs

½ cup of melted ghee

1 cup of bacon bits

3 cups of almond flour

Directions

Preheat the oven to about 350 degrees F.

In a bowl melt ghee, then mix bacon bits, lemon thyme, eggs, baking soda and almond flour until well combined.

Place the mixture in a muffin pan lined with muffin liners and bake for about 18 to 20 minutes.

Nutritional information per serving:

Calories 300, Fat 28 g, Carbs 7 g, Protein 11 g

Keto Bread Snacks

Keto Soft Pretzel

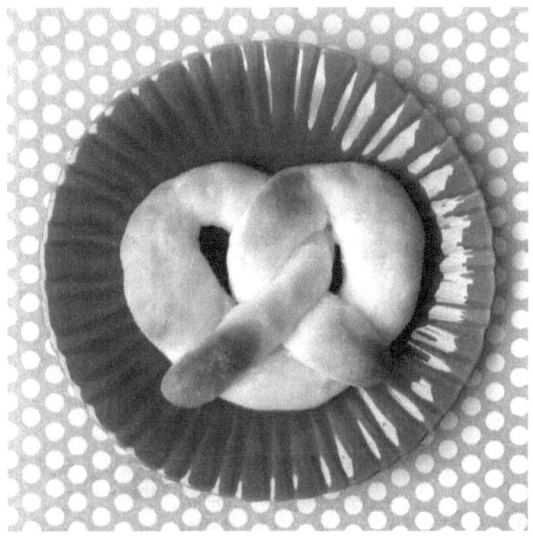

Prep time: 15 Minutes

Cook time: 14 Minutes

Total time: 29 Minutes

Servings: makes 6 pretzels

Ingredients

5 tablespoons of cream cheese

3 cups of mozzarella cheese, shredded

3 large eggs, divided

1 teaspoon of onion powder

1 teaspoon of garlic powder

1 tablespoon baking powder

2 cups of almond flour blanched

Coarse sea salt

Directions

Preheat the oven to about 425 degrees F then line a baking dish with silpat or some parchment paper.

In a bowl, mix onion powder, garlic powder, baking powder and almond flour; combine until well mixed.

In a bowl, whisk one egg, you will use this as egg wash for the upper part of pretzels. The remaining eggs will be used in making the dough.

In a microwave-safe bowl, mix cream cheese and mozzarella cheese then place in a microwave. Microwave for around one minute and 30 seconds then remove and mix well. Return the mixture to the microwave for another one minute then remove and mix again until combined well.

In the bowl with almond flour mix, add eggs and mix well making sure the ingredients are incorporated well. If the dough is very stringy, place back in microwave for another 30 seconds to make it soft and combine again.

Divide equally the dough into 6 portions then roll every portion into the shape of a bread stick and fold them into a pretzel. Using the egg wash, brush the upper part of every pretzel. Sprinkle with some salt on top then bake for about 12-14 minutes until they are golden brown.

Serve with some nacho cheese sauce or spicy mustard.

Nutritional information per serving:

Calories 449, Fat 35.5 g, Protein 27.8 g, Carbs 10 g

Keto Croutons

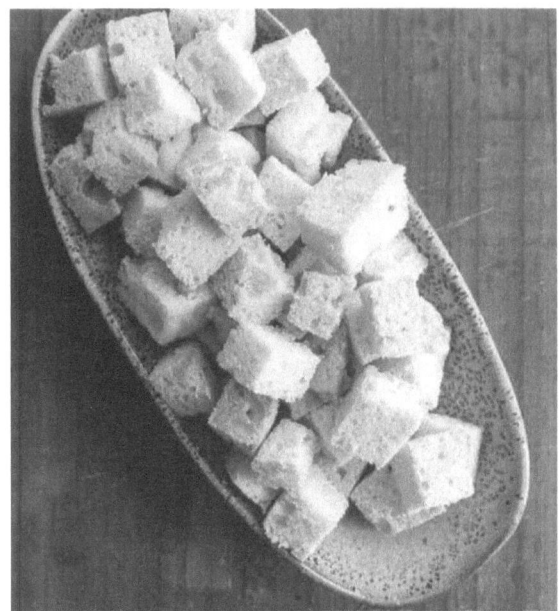

Prep time: 5 Minutes

Cook time: 5 Minutes

Total time: 10 Minutes

Servings: 4

Ingredients

2 ½ tablespoons of coconut oil

1 whisked egg

1 teaspoon of Italian seasoning

Pinch of salt

½ teaspoon of baking powder

1/3 cup of almond flour

Directions

Preheat the oven to about 300 degrees F or 150 degrees C.

Mix all the ingredients in a bowl, and then transfer it to a microwave safe dish or container and microwave for about 90 seconds on high speed. The time may be different depending on the type of microwave you have.

Leave to cool then remove from the dish and cut into small pieces. Spread the pieces on a baking dish and toast for about 8-10 minutes in the oven until crunchy and browned.

Nutritional information per serving:

Calories 135, Fat 14 g, Carbs 2 g, Protein 3 g

Keto Bread Twists

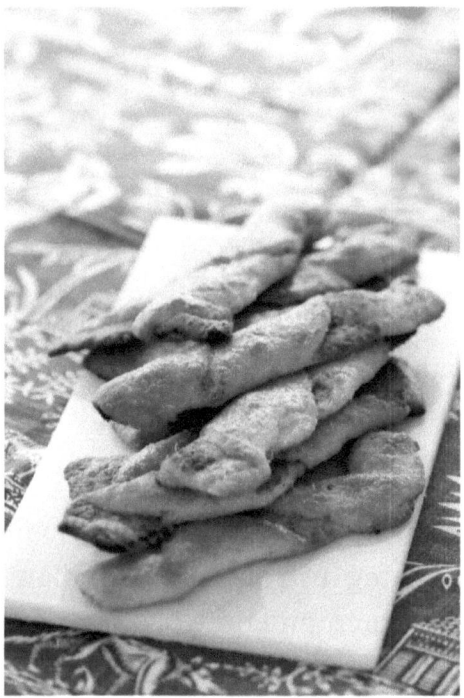

Prep time: 10 Minutes

Cook time: 20 Minutes

Total time: 30 Minutes

Servings: 10

Ingredients

1 egg for brushing the top of bread twists

2 ounces of green pesto

1 egg

2 2/3 ounces of butter

1 ½ cups of cheese shredded

1 teaspoon of baking powder

½ teaspoon of salt

4 tablespoons of coconut flour

½ cup of almond flour

Directions

Preheat the oven to about 175 degrees Celsius.

Mix all the dry ingredients in a medium bowl.

In a pan over low heat, mix the cheese and butter using a wooden fork and stir until butter becomes smooth. Once smooth, crack the egg and mix well. Mix in the dry ingredients and combine well to form dough.

Put dough in the middle of 2 sheets of parchment paper and make a rectangle shape around 1/5 inch thick using a rolling pin. Remove the upper part of parchment paper, and add pesto on top and slice into one inch pieces.

Transfer them onto a baking sheet lined with parchment paper and brush them with the egg wash. Put in the oven for 15 to 20 minutes or until golden brown.

Keto Diet Snacks

Nutritional information per serving:

Calories 204, Protein 7 g, Fat 18 g, Carbs 1 g

Keto Bread Sticks

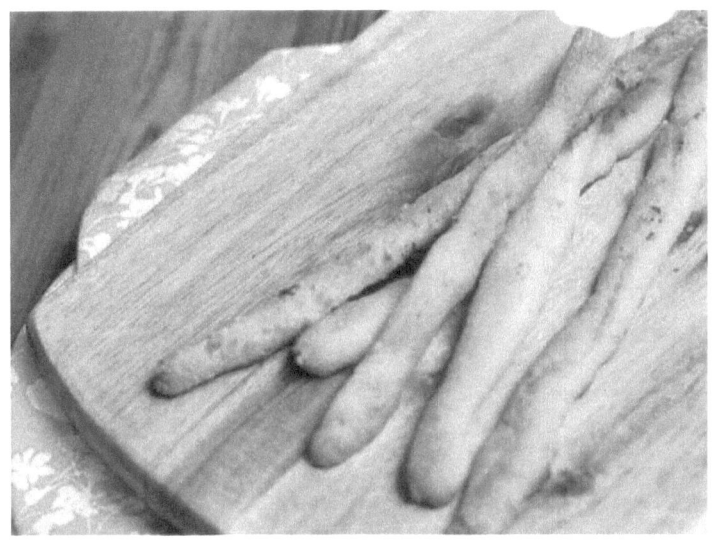

Prep time: 10 Minutes

Cook time: 10 Minutes

Total time: 20 Minutes

Servings: 20

Ingredients

1 tablespoon of dried parsley

1 teaspoon of rosemary, dried

1 tablespoon of crushed garlic

1 medium egg

Pinch of salt

2 tablespoons of full fat cream cheese

85 grams of almond meal

170 grams of mozzarella, grated

Directions

Mix salt, almond flour, cream cheese, shredded cheese and the seasonings in a microwave safe dish. Microwave for one minute on high speed, mix then microwave for thirty seconds on high speed, add in egg and stir slowly to create cheesy mixture.

Roll small pieces of mozzarella dough into thin bread sticks and place on a lined baking sheet. Bake for about ten minutes at 220 degrees Celsius until browned. Depending on the thickness, cooking time may vary.

Nutritional information per serving:

Calories 58, Fat 4.9 g, Carbs 1.2 g, Protein 3.1 g

Keto Crackers

Keto Graham Crackers

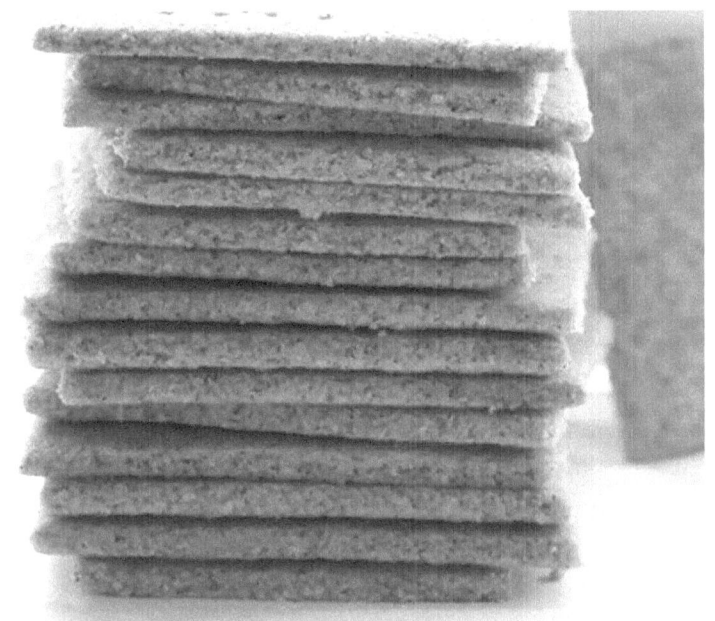

Prep time: 15 Minutes

Cook time: 50 Minutes

Total time: 1 Hour 5 Minutes

Servings: 10

Ingredients

1 teaspoon of vanilla extract

2 teaspoons of Yacon syrup

2 tablespoons of melted butter

1 egg

Pinch of salt

1 teaspoon of baking powder

2 teaspoons of cinnamon

1/3 cup of swerve sweetener

2 cups of almond flour

Directions

Preheat the oven to about 300 degrees F.

In a medium bowl, mix salt, baking powder, cinnamon, sweetener and almond flour. Mix in vanilla extract, yacon syrup, melted butter and egg. Mix well until a dough begins to form.

Place the dough on a parchment paper and make into a rough rectangle then put another parchment paper onto the dough. Using a rolling pin, roll the dough as equally as possible to around ¼ or 1/8 inch thickness.

Remove the top sheet of parchment paper and with a pizza wheel or sharp knife cut the dough into squares of around 2*2 inches. Transfer the scored dough together with the parchment paper to a baking sheet and bake for around 20-30 minutes until firm and brown.

Remove the baking sheet from the oven and let the crackers to cool for around 30 minutes then break up the dough along the score lines.

Return to the oven making sure the oven is off, however if the oven is very cool turn it back on and set it to nothing more than 200 degrees F. Let the crackers stay in the oven for another 30 minutes then remove from oven and leave them to cool completely.

Nutritional information per serving:

Calories 156, Fat 13.35 g, Carbs 6.21 g, Protein 5.21 g

Keto Crackers

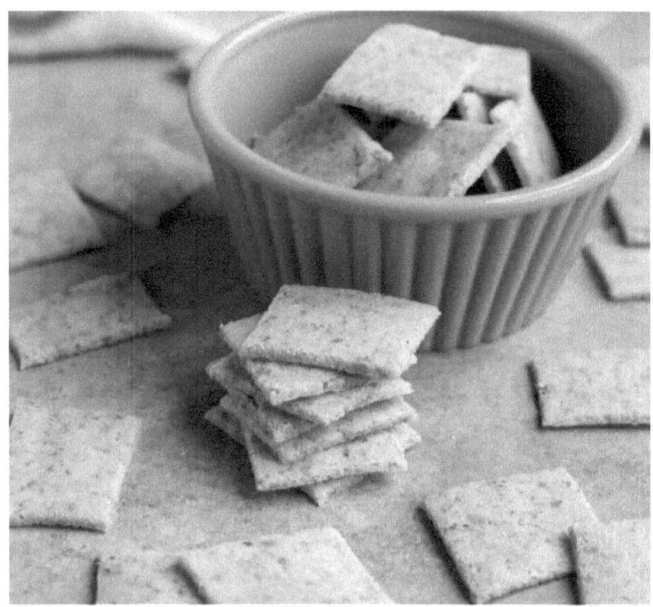

Prep time: 10 Minutes

Cook time: 15 Minutes

Total time: 25 Minutes

Servings: 6

Ingredients

1 tablespoon of coconut oil

2 tablespoons of water

¾ teaspoon of sea salt

1 tablespoon of flax meal

2 tablespoons of sunflower seeds

1 cup of almond flour

Directions

Preheat the oven to about 350 degrees F.

Mix salt, psyllium, sunflower seeds and almond flour in a food processor. Add coconut oil and water, and mix until dough is formed.

Place the dough on a parchment paper then press it flat. Put a parchment paper on top of the dough and roll to around 1/8 inch thick.

Remove the top parchment paper and place on a chopping board, slice into an inch squares then sprinkle with some salt on top if you like.

Put the sliced dough in a baking dish, bake until golden brown at 350 degrees F. Let them cool on a wire rack and enjoy.

Nutritional information per serving:

Calories 151, Fat 13 g, Carbs 6 g Protein 4 g

Keto Seed Crackers

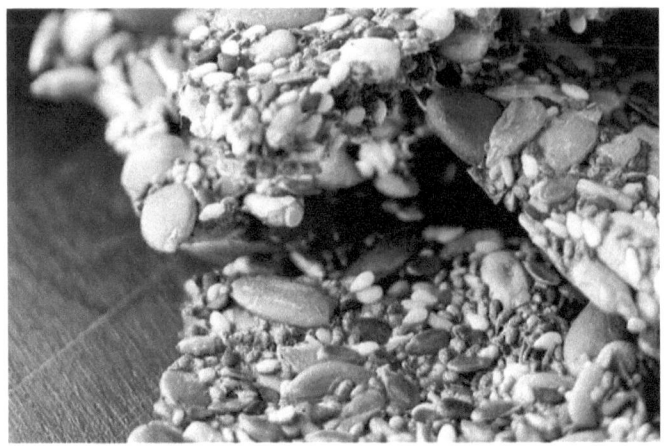

Prep time: 15 Minutes

Cook time: 1 Hour

Total time: 1 Hour 15 Minutes

Servings: 10

Ingredients

1 teaspoon of chilli flakes

1 tablespoon of thyme

1 ½ cups of water

1 teaspoon of salt

¼ cup of flax seed

½ cup of sesame seeds

¾ cup of pumpkin seeds

1 cup of sunflower seeds

Directions

Preheat the oven to about 340 degrees F.

In a bowl, mix all the ingredients for about 10-15 minutes until the seeds soak in the water. Mix well, then divide equally the mixture between two lined baking trays and evenly spread. The thickness should be around 3-4 millimeters. If the mixture is very thick they will turn out to be seed cookies, if they are thin the crackers will be extremely fragile.

Bake for around 1 hour rotating the baking trays about halfway through the time. If the crackers are not crispy after one hour, place back in the oven for 5-10 more minutes.

Remove from oven and leave them to cool; if you would like to store them do so in an airtight container.

Nutritional information per serving:

Calories 192, Fat 15.4 g, Carbs 9.1 g, Protein 7.5 g

Keto Cheesy Crackers

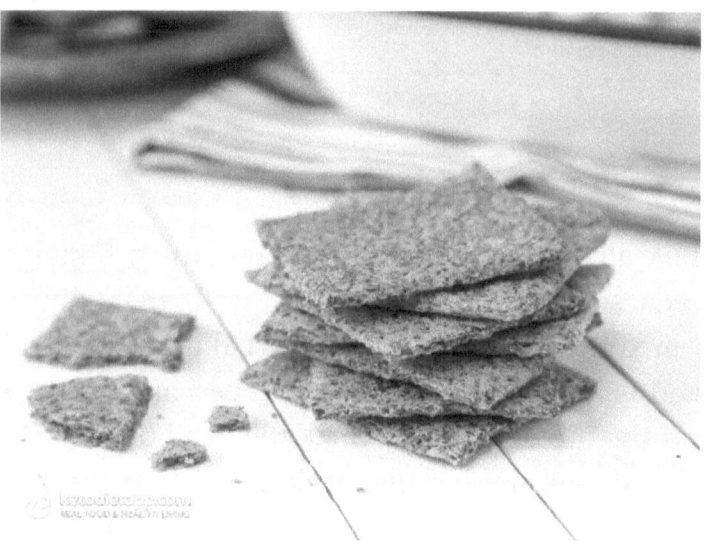

Prep time: 20 Minutes

Cook time: 40 Minutes

Total time: 60 Minutes

Servings: 32 crackers

Ingredients

1 cup of water

¼ teaspoon of black pepper

1 teaspoon of salt

1 cup of parmesan cheese, grated

2 tablespoons of whole psyllium husks

½ cup of flax meal

1 cup of almond flour

Directions

Mix pepper, salt, psyllium and almond flour. Once well mixed, add in the parmesan cheese and mix again. Add in water then with a spatula or your hands combine well. Let the dough sit for around 10-15 minutes.

In the meantime, preheat the oven to around 320 degrees F or 160 degrees C and equally divide dough into two equal portions.

Put one of the portions on top of parchment paper then parchment paper on top of dough. Roll the dough until it is extremely thin around 1/8 inch. With the sides of parchment paper fold over the dough from sides then using a rolling pin, roll the dough again. Slice dough into 16 equal cuts using pizza cutter or knife.

Repeat the same for the other half portion of dough that was put aside. Bake for around 40-45 minutes then if you like, you can serve with guacamole or marinara sauce. You can use silicon mat, as the crackers tend to stick on the parchment paper.

Store up to 5 days at room temp or place in the freezer for 3 months.

Nutritional Information per serving:

Calories 168, Carbs 6.3 g, Protein 8.4 g Protein, Fat 13.4 g

Fat Head Crackers

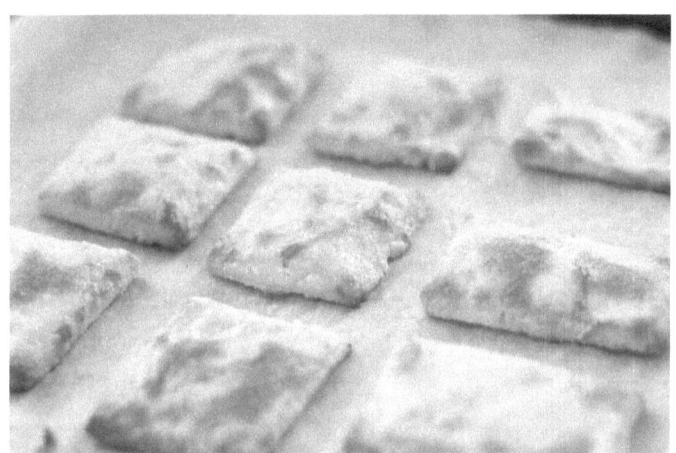

Prep time: 10 Minutes

Cook time: 10 Minutes

Total time: 20 Minutes

Servings: 6

Ingredients

½ teaspoon of vanilla extract

Salt to taste

1 egg

2 tablespoons of cream cheese

85 grams of almond flour

170 grams of shredded mozzarella

Directions

Mix in a microwave safe bowl, almond flour and shredded cheese. Microwave on high heat for about one minute, mix then microwave the mixture again on high heat for 30 more seconds. Add in the remaining ingredients and gently mix.

Put the dough between two parchment papers then thinly roll using a rolling pin. Remove top parchment paper and if the dough is hard and very difficult to use, place it back in microwave for around 10-20 seconds to become soft but make sure not to place it for long as it might cook the egg.

Slice dough into small pieces and put each piece on a lined baking sheet. Bake for around 5 minutes on every side at 220 degrees C or until crisp and browned.

Cool the crackers on a rack and place in a dish that is airtight then put in the fridge. You can store the airtight container in the pantry for 3 days if weather is quite cool.

Nutritional information per serving:

Calories 203, Fat 16.8 g, Carbs 4g, Protein 11g

Keto Chips

Zucchini Chips

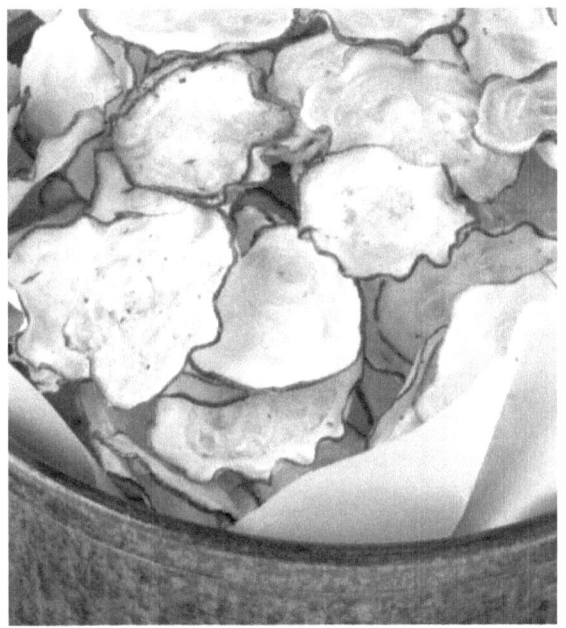

Prep time: 15 Minutes

Cook time: 12 Hours

Total time: 12 Hours 15 Minutes

Servings: 8

Ingredients

2 teaspoons of sea salt, coarse

2 tablespoons of white balsamic vinegar

2 tablespoons of extra virgin olive oil

4 cups of sliced thinly zucchini

Directions

Chop very tiny zucchini slices using a mandolin.

Mix vinegar and olive oil in a bowl. Add in the zucchini and mix with the olive oil and vinegar.

Place zucchini in a dehydrator then add salt. The drying period may differ between 8-14 hours depending on the thinness of the zucchini.

You can also prepare in the oven. Line a baking tray with parchment paper, and then place the zucchini on top. Bake for around 2-3 hours at 200 degrees Celsius. Make sure to turn ½ way while cooking. Once ready, store in an airtight container.

Nutritional information per serving:

Calories 40, Fat 3.6 g, Carbs 2.3 g, Protein 0.7 g

Radish Chips

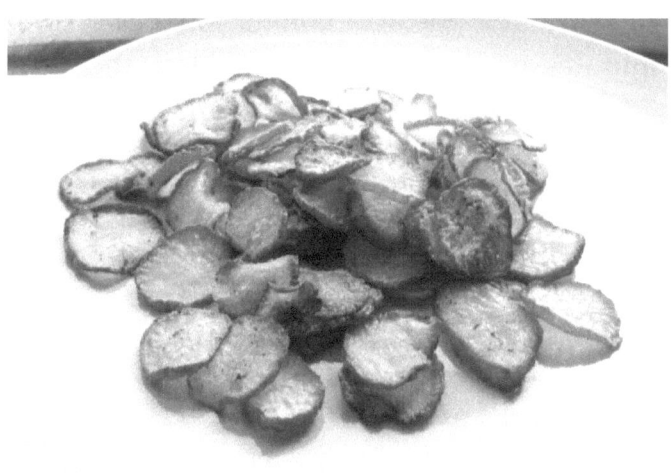

Prep time: 10 Minutes

Cook time: 10 Minutes

Total time: 20 Minutes

Servings: 4

Ingredients

½ teaspoon of sea salt

16 ounces of radishes

Olive oil for deep-frying

Directions

Heat oil in a frying pan to about 325 degrees F.

Slice radishes into tiny slices using a sharp knife or mandolin. Put radishes in a pot with boiling water and cook for about 4-5 minutes or until the skins lighten and turn translucent.

Put the radishes in a colander to drain the water. Fry the radishes in hot oil for about 8-10 minutes or until golden brown.

Nutritional information per serving:

Calories 48, Fat 4.7 g, Carbs 2.4 g, Protein 0.8 g

Keto Cheese Chips

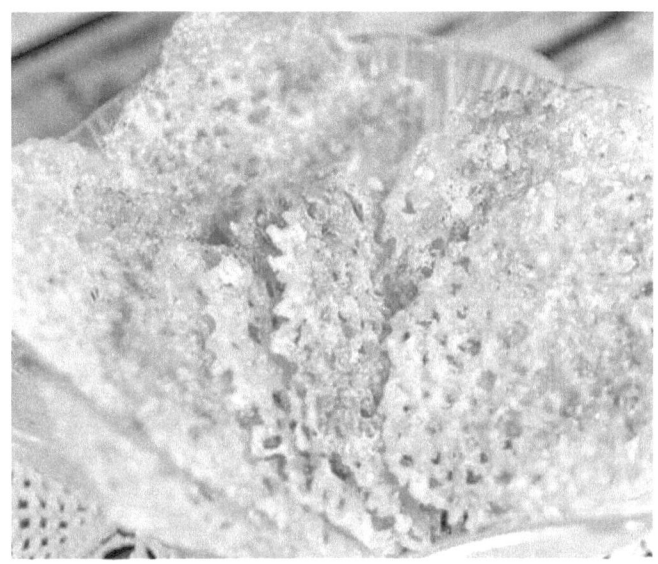

Prep time: 5 Minutes

Cook time: 6 Minutes

Total time: 11 Minutes

Servings: 2

Ingredients

1 pinch of paprika

3 slices of cheddar cheese

Directions

Preheat the oven to 375 degrees F.

Slice cheese into quarters and place them on a lined baking sheet ensuring that you leave adequate space between them. Sprinkle with paprika and bake for 6 minutes or until golden brown.

Use a paper towel to get rid of any excess oil..

Nutritional information per serving:

Calories 225, Fat 21 g, Carbs 0 g, Protein 16 g

Keto Salami Chips

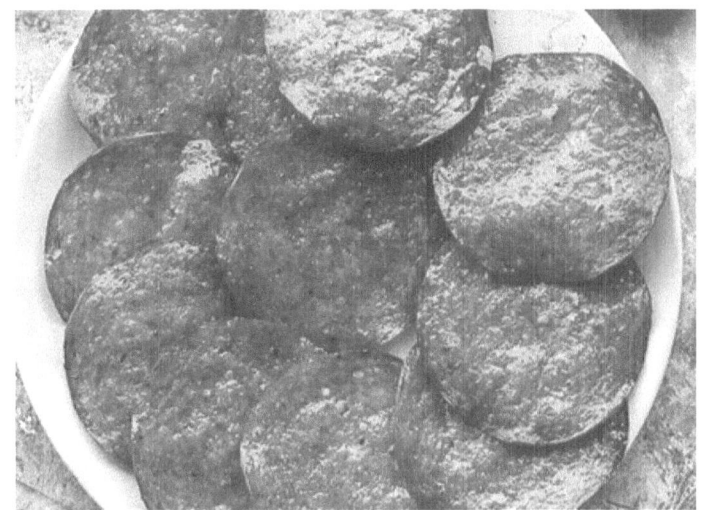

Prep Time: 5 Minutes

Cook Time: 20 Minutes

Total Time: 25 Minutes

Servings: 2

Ingredients

1 teaspoon of olive oil

3.5 ounces sliced salami

Directions

Preheat the oven to 355 degrees F.

Put the slices of salami on a baking dish lined with parchment paper. Drizzle some olive oil and let them cook for about 15 to 25 minutes.

You may also microwave the slices on high speed for around 2 minutes over a paper towel to ensure fast crispiness.

Nutritional Information per Serving:

Calories 147, Fat 13 g, Carbs 1 g, Protein 7 g

Keto Pepperoni Chips

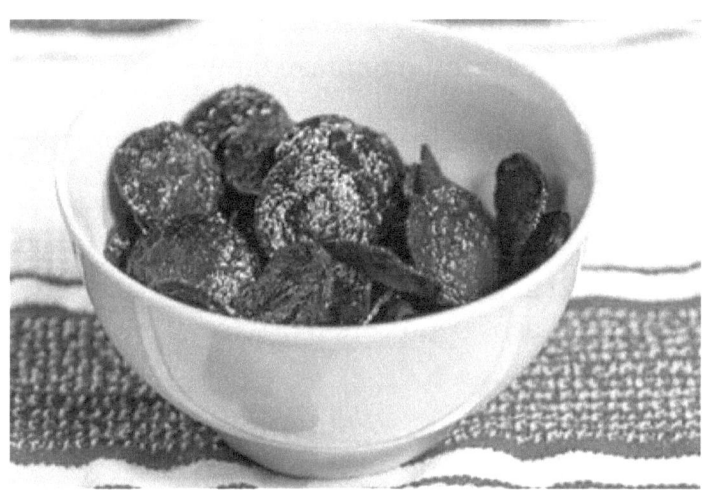

Prep time: 2 Minutes

Cook time: 6 Minutes

Total time: 8 Minutes

Servings: 6

Ingredients

6 ounces of thinly sliced Pepperoni

Directions

Preheat the oven to 400 degrees F.

Line a baking tray with parchment paper and put the sliced pepperoni in one on the baking sheet.

Bake for around 5 minutes, remove from the oven and pat off the extra oil using paper towel. Place the slices back in the oven and bake for another minute to make them crispier.

Once ready, remove the slices from oven and place on paper towels for about 2 minutes, enjoy.

Nutritional Information per Serving:

Calories 130, Fat 12 g, Carbs 0 g, Protein 6 g

Keto Nuts

Keto Spiced Pecans

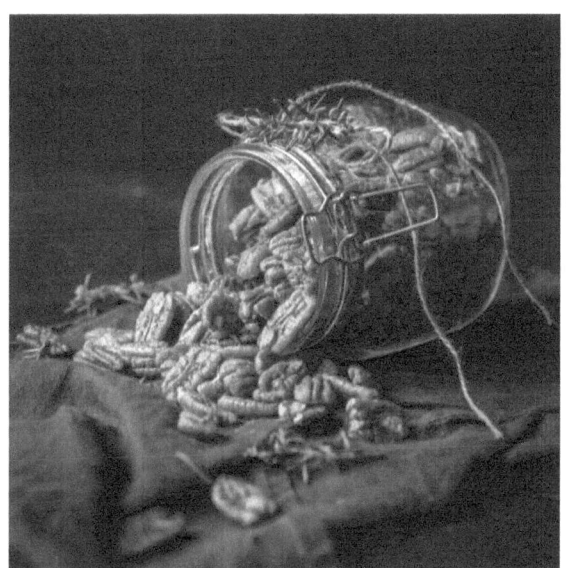

Prep time: 5 Minutes

Cook time: 15 Minutes

Total time: 20 Minutes

Servings: 8

Ingredients

¼ cup of extra virgin oil

2 teaspoons of fresh lemon zest

2 teaspoons of salt, pink Himalayan

¼ teaspoon of smoked paprika

¼ teaspoon of onion powder

¼ teaspoon of garlic powder

4 tablespoons of fresh rosemary, copped roughly

4 cups of pecans

¼ teaspoon of cayenne pepper, optional

Directions

Preheat the oven to about 355 degrees F or 180 degrees C.

Put the pecans into a bowl. Add in spices apart from lemon zest, add in olive oil and mix well until combined and the pecans are well and evenly coated.

Pour the coated pecans onto a baking tray and spread them in one layer then bake for about 10-15 minutes until they are toasty and golden. Be careful and watch the nuts at about the last half of their cooking time to avoid burning.

Remove from the oven and leave them to slightly cool then sprinkle the lemon zest over and mix. Let the nuts completely cool then place in airtight containers.

Nutritional information per serving:

Calories 348, Carbs 7.3 g, Protein 4.6 g, Fat 36.1 g

Dill Pickle Almonds

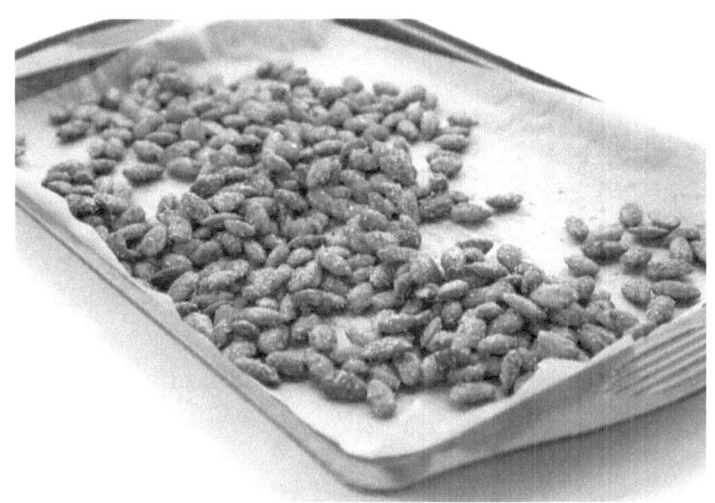

Prep time: 10 Minutes

Cook time: 12 Minutes

Total time: 22 Minutes

Servings: 12

Ingredients

¼ teaspoon of coriander

½ teaspoon of pepper

¾ teaspoon of garlic powder

2 teaspoons of dried dill

2 teaspoons of salt

2 teaspoon of citric acid

3 cups of almonds

1 egg white

Directions

Preheat the oven to about 350 degrees F and line a baking dish with some parchment paper.

In a bowl, mix the egg until it becomes frothy then mix in almonds making sure they are coated well.

Sprinkle the coriander, pepper, garlic, dill, salt and citric acid, tossing to mix well.

Bake for 10-12 minutes or until the almonds turn brown then allow them to cool, enjoy.

Nutritional information per serving:

Calories 207, Fat 17.05 g, Carbs 7.93 g, Protein 7.61 g

Almond Cranberry Trail Mix

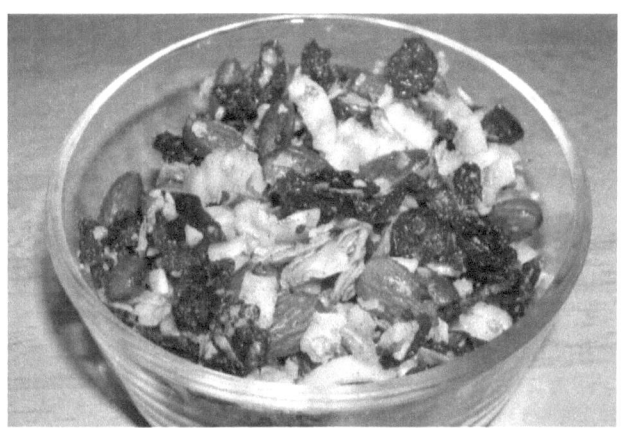

Prep time: 10 Minutes

Cook time: 1 Hour 8 Minutes

Total time: 1 Hour 18 Minutes

Servings: 12

Ingredients

½ teaspoon of salt

½ teaspoon of ground cinnamon

½ of swerve

1 egg white

1 cup of dried cranberries, sugar free

1 cup of flaked coconut, unsweetened

1 cup of whole almonds, raw

Directions

Preheat the oven to about 350 degrees F then evenly spread the almonds on a baking dish.

Bake for around 8 minutes until the nuts become slightly darker then completely cool.

Lower the heat to around 225 degrees F then in a mixing bowl mix cranberries, coconut and almonds. In another bowl, whisk the egg until it becomes foamy.

Add into the almond mixture the egg mixture and mix well then in another bowl mix salt, cinnamon and sweetener. Add into almond mixture and combine again.

Spread the coated almonds on a baking dish greased with some oil. Bake as you stir frequently for about 15 minutes. Once ready, cool completely and store in an airtight container.

Nutritional information per serving:

Calories 140, Fat 9 g, Carbs 5 g, Protein 3 g

Keto Roll Up Recipes

Hot Dogs In A Blanket

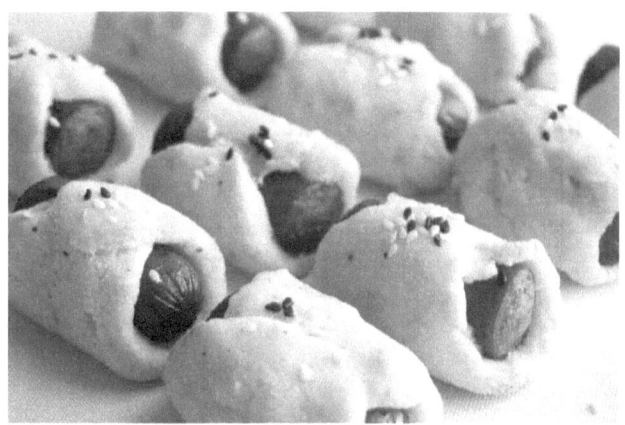

Prep time: 10 Minutes

Cook time: 20 Minutes

Total time: 30 Minutes

Servings: 12

Ingredients

½ teaspoon of sesame seeds

½ teaspoon of pink salt

¼ teaspoon of garlic powder

¼ teaspoon of baking powder

1 egg

Keto Diet Snacks

¾ cup of almond flour

½ cup of mozzarella cheese, shredded

4 hot dogs, medium size

Directions

Microwave mozzarella then once melted, add in egg and almond flour, and mix well until combined.

Slice hot dog to three equal portions and put aside. Mix into the flour mixture salt, garlic and baking powder until well combined then with your hands knead the dough.

Divide the dough into small twelve equal parts and put them on a parchment paper lined baking dish.

Put each of the hot dog pieces into dough and roll up like blanket. Sprinkle with some sesame seeds and press them down into the dough. Bake for around 17-20 minutes at 350 degrees F.

Once ready, let it cool, then enjoy.

Nutritional information per serving:

Calories 332.25, Fat 27.5 g, Carbs 7.25 g, Protein 16.25 g

Artichoke Dip Jalapeno Poppers

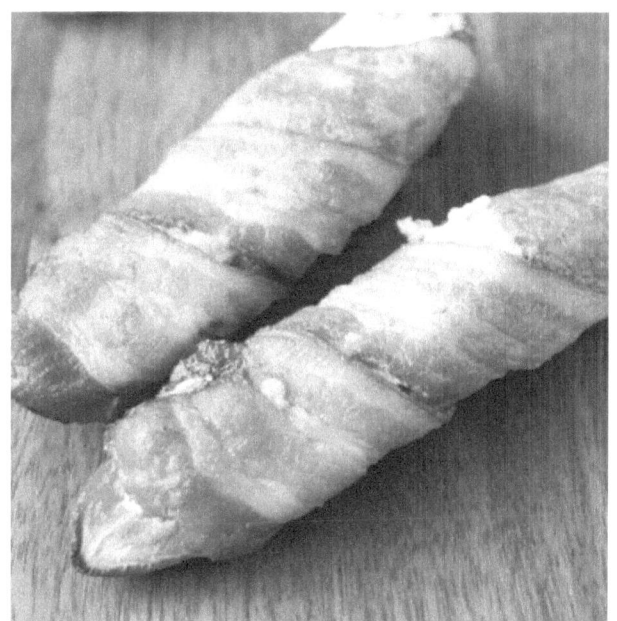

Prep time: 20 Minutes

Cook time: 30 Minutes

Total time: 50 Minutes

Servings: 12 poppers

Ingredients

12 slices of bacon

6 large jalapenos

Salt to taste

Keto Diet Snacks

1/8 teaspoon of garlic powder

¼ teaspoon of chili powder

¼ cup of shredded cheese

1 tablespoon of white onion, chopped finely

¼ cup of mayo

4 ounces of cubed cream cheese

3 ounces of canned artichokes, drained and copped

Directions

Preheat the oven to around 400 degrees F.

In a microwave-safe bowl, add in the cream cheese and artichokes. Microwave the mixture for around 30-45 seconds until the cheese melts then mix well. Put in some salt, garlic, chili powder, cheese, onion and mayo then combine until well mixed.

Slice in half the jalapenos and get rid of the seeds and veins. Rinse the jalapenos then scoop around one tablespoon of the cheese mixture and put into the jalapeno well. You might need less cheese mixture in case of small jalapenos.

Wrap using bacon each of the stuffed jalapenos and put on baking sheet then bake for about 30 minutes until the bacon becomes crispy and the jalapenos are tender. You might have to use lesser time when you are using thin bacon or small jalapenos. You can look at the jalapenos after around 15 minutes to see how long you will need to continue cooking them.

Nutritional information per serving:

Calories 146, Fat 11.6 g, Carbs 3.6 g, Protein 5.7 g

Steak Fajita Roll-Ups

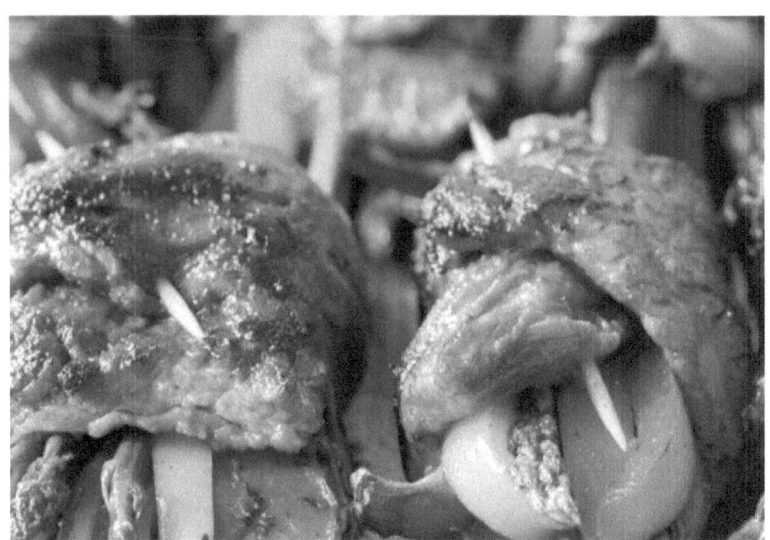

Prep time: 15 Minutes

Cook time: 15 Minutes

Total time: 30 Minutes

Servings: 12

Ingredients

Taco sauce

2 tablespoons of olive oil

1 packet of fajita seasoning mix

1 red onion

1 bunch of baby asparagus

2 bell peppers

1 ½ pounds of flank steak

Directions

Using a knife, chop the steak along the edge, as chopping the steak parallel makes it easy to open like a book with 2 layers. Stretch the steak and cover it using a transparent film. Using a rolling pin pound the steak until it becomes thin. Remove the film and add fajita seasoning on both sides. Slice the steak into 12 sections of about 2.5*5 inches.

Seed and cut the bell peppers into tinny strips, cut the ends of asparagus ensuring that the asparagus tops are of the same length like bell peppers, throw away ends. Peel and slice the onion.

Heat a pan over high heat. Once the pan is hot, add in onions, asparagus and the peppers. Heat them for about two minutes for each batch and remove ensuring that the peppers have char marks.

Reduce the temperature to medium, place several onion cuts, asparagus spears and pepper strips across every steak strip making cross arrangement. Fold the steak edges tightly round vegetables and pin the ends with a toothpick.

In a pan over medium heat add one tablespoon of cooking oil then add six rolls in the pan. Let them cook for two minutes per side and then turn. Repeat the same for the remaining rolls then serve.

Nutritional Information per serving:

Calories 106, Fat 5 g, Carbs 1 g, Protein 12 g

Keto Mummy Dogs

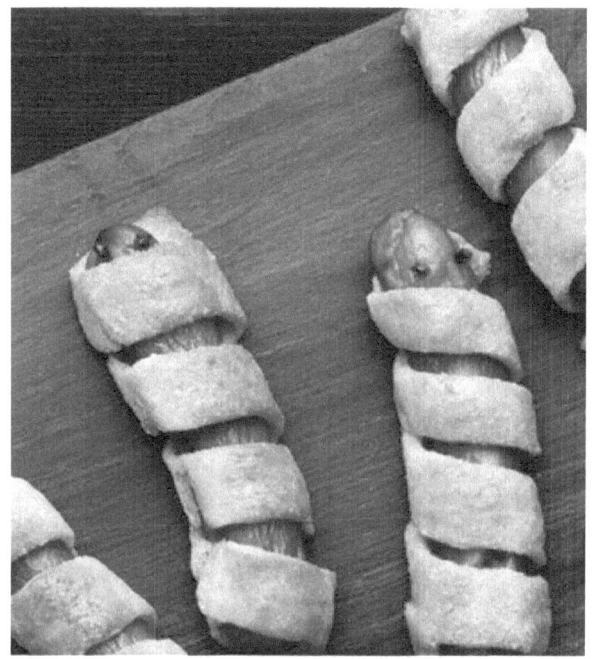

Prep time: 25 Minutes

Cook time: 20 Minutes

Total time: 45 Minutes

Servings: 4

Ingredients

16 cloves to be used as mummies eyes

1 egg to brush the dough

1 pound of sausages

Keto Diet Snacks

1 egg

1 ½ cups of shredded cheese

2 2/3 ounces of butter

1 teaspoon of baking powder

½ teaspoon of salt

4 tablespoons of coconut flour

½ cup of almond flour

Directions

Preheat the oven to about 175 degrees Celsius.

In a bowl, mix baking powder, coconut flour and almond flour.

Heat cheese and butter in a skillet over low heat. Mix using a wooden spoon for a few minutes until the cheese mixture is smooth. Remove from heat and crack an egg into the mixture and mix.

Add in the flour mixture and combine to form dough. Compress the dough into rectangle of about 8 by 14 inches. Slice into eight long pieces not wide than 1.5 to 2 cm inches.

Wrap the hot dog in the dough and brush with egg. Put on a baking sheet lined with parchment paper and place in the oven for 15 to 20 minutes or until golden brown.

Place 2 cloves on the hot dog for decoration but do not eat.

Nutritional information per serving:

Calories 746, Protein 29 g, Fat 68 g, Carbs 7 g

Keto Cheese Roll-Ups

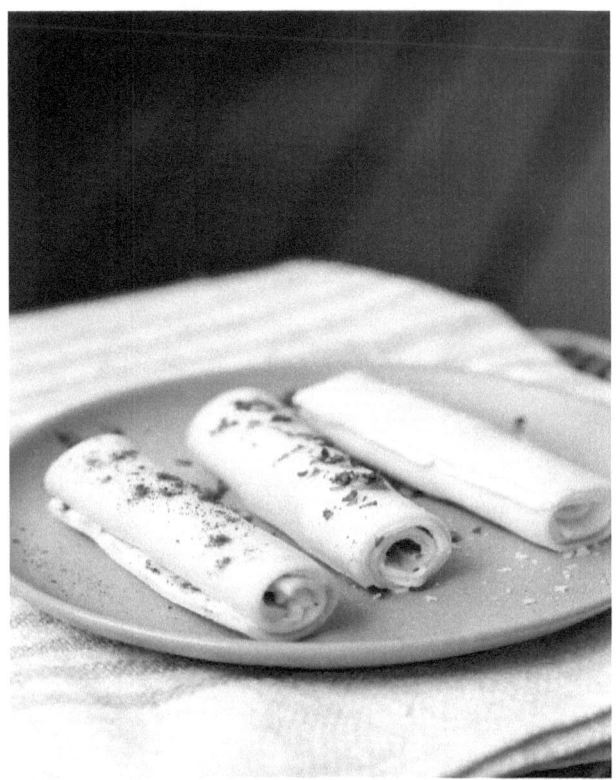

Prep time: 5 Minutes

Cook time: 0 Minutes

Total time: 5 Minutes

Servings: 4

Ingredients

2 ounces of butter

8 ounces of sliced provolone cheese

Directions

Put cheese pieces on a chopping board. Slice the butter into thin portions using a knife or cheese slicer. Cover each cheese slice using butter then roll up. Enjoy

Nutritional information per serving:

Calories 335, Carbs 2g, Fat 31g, Protein 13g

Conclusion

Thank you again for downloading this book!

I hope you now know some snack recipes that you can prepare to eat even as you start or continue with your ketogenic diet journey.

What you need to do now is to try out these tasty recipes and you will be amazed at how good they are.

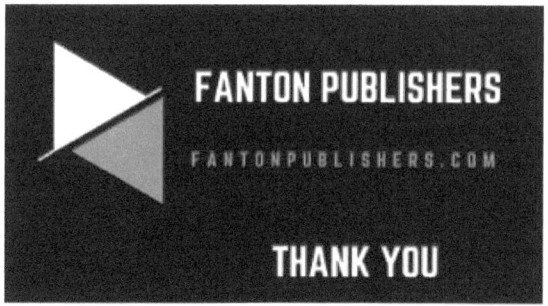

Do You Like My Book & Approach To Publishing?

If you like my writing and style and would love the ease of learning literally everything you can get your hands on from Fantonpublishers.com, I'd really need you to do me either of the following favors.

1: First, I'd Love It If You Leave a Review of This Book on Amazon.

2: Check Out My Other Keto Diet Books

KETOGENIC DIET: Keto Diet Made Easy: Beginners Guide on How to Burn Fat Fast With the Keto Diet (Including 100+ Recipes That You Can Prepare Within 20 Minutes)- New Edition

KETOGENIC DIET: Ketogenic Diet Recipes That You Can Prepare Using 7 Ingredients and Less in Less Than 30 Minutes

Ketogenic Diet: With A Sustainable Twist: Lose Weight Rapidly With Ketogenic Diet Recipes You Can Make Within 25 Minutes

Ketogenic Diet: Keto Diet Breakfast Recipes

Fat Bombs: Keto Fat Bombs: 50+ Savory and Sweet Ketogenic Diet Fat Bombs That You MUST Prepare Before Any Other!

Snacks: Keto Diet Snacks: 50+ Savory and Sweet Ketogenic Diet Snacks That You MUST Prepare Before Any Other!

Desserts: Keto Diet Desserts: 50+ Savory and Sweet Ketogenic Diet Desserts That You MUST Prepare Before Any Other!

Ketogenic Diet: Ketogenic Diet Lunch and Dinner Recipes

Ketogenic Diet: Keto Diet Cookbook For Vegetarians

Ketogenic Diet: Ketogenic Slow Cooker Cookbook: Keto Slow Cooker Recipes That You Can Prepare Using 7 Ingredients Or Less

Note: This list may not represent all my Keto diet books. You can check the full list by visiting my Author Central: amazon.com/author/fantonpublishers or my website http://www.fantonpublishers.com

Get updates when we publish any book on the Ketogenic diet: http://bit.ly/2fantonpubketo

Closely related to the keto diet is intermittent fasting. I also publish books on Intermittent Fasting.

One of the books is shown below:

Intermittent Fasting: A Complete Beginners Guide to Intermittent Fasting For Weight Loss, Increased Energy, and A Healthy Life

Get updates when we publish any book on intermittent fasting: http://bit.ly/2fantonbooksIF

To get a list of all my other books, please fantonwriters.com, my author central or let me send you the list by requesting them below: http://bit.ly/2fantonpubnewbooks

3: Let's Get In Touch

Antony

Website: http://www.fantonpublishers.com/

Email: Support@fantonpublishers.com

Twitter: https://twitter.com/FantonPublisher

Facebook Page: https://www.facebook.com/Fantonpublisher/

My Ketogenic Diet Books Page: https://www.facebook.com/pg/Fast-Keto-Meals-336338180266944

Private Facebook Group For Readers: https://www.facebook.com/groups/FantonPublishers/

Pinterest: https://www.pinterest.com/fantonpublisher/

4: Grab Some Freebies On Your Way Out; Giving Is Receiving, Right?

I gave you 2 freebies at the start of the book, one on general life transformation and one about the Ketogenic diet. Grab them here if you didn't grab them earlier.

Ketogenic Diet Freebie: http://bit.ly/2fantonpubketo

5 Pillar Life Transformation Checklist: http://bit.ly/2fantonfreebie

5: Suggest Topics That You'd Love Me To Cover To Increase Your Knowledge Bank.

I am looking forward to seeing your suggestions and insights; you could even suggest improvements to this book. Simply send me a message on Support@fantonpublishers.com.

PSS: Let Me Also Help You Save Some Money!

If you are a heavy reader, have you considered subscribing to Kindle Unlimited? You can read this and millions of other books for just $9.99 a month)! You can check it out by searching for Kindle Unlimited on Amazon!

www.ingramcontent.com/pod-product-compliance
Lightning Source LLC
Chambersburg PA
CBHW030154100526
44592CB00009B/274